T0090134

ACQUAINTED WITH THE NIGHT

ACQUAINTED

WITH
THE
Night

a parent's quest to understand depression
and bipolar disorder in his children

PAUL RAEBURN

BROADWAY BOOKS   NEW YORK

Visit our website at www.broadwaybooks.com

First trade paperback edition published 2005.

Book design by Ellen Cipriano

Excerpt from "Acquainted with the Night" from *The Poetry of Robert Frost*, edited by Edward Connery Lathem. Copyright © 1928, 1969 by Henry Holt and Company, copyright © 1956 by Robert Frost. Reprinted by permission of Henry Holt and Company, LLC.

The Library of Congress has cataloged the hardcover edition as:

Raeburn, Paul, 1950–
  Acquainted with the night : a parent's quest to understand depression and bipolar disorder in his children / Paul Raeburn.—1st ed.
    p. cm.
  1. Raeburn, Paul, 1950—Family. 2. Raeburn, Alex—Mental health.
3. Raeburn, Alicia—Mental health. 4. Raeburn family. 5. Depression in children—Patients—United States—Biography. 6. Manic-depressive illness in children—Patients—United States—Biography. I. Title.

RJ506.D4R34 2004
618.92'8527'0092—dc22
[B]   2003063788

ISBN-13: 978-0-7679-1438-3

To Alex and Alicia

I have been one acquainted with the night
I have walked out in the rain—and back in rain.
I have outwalked the furthest city light.
I have looked down the saddest city lane.
. . . I have been one acquainted with the night.

—ROBERT FROST

t is an unusually chilly night in April. I am driving fast on a dark, nearly deserted highway, in an unfamiliar place, struggling to keep up with an ambulance in the headlights in front of me. My hands are steady enough if I grip the wheel hard. The ambulance is headed toward a psychiatric hospital forty miles from my home. My son, Alex, eleven years old, is inside, strapped to a gurney and bound at the hands and feet.

This morning, in school, Alex was told that the scheduled fifth-grade art lesson had been canceled. Something detonated inside him. He became enraged. He screamed at his teacher, and ran from the classroom. She called out to him, demanding that he return, but he kept running. He fled blindly down the hallway, smashing the glass face of a large wall clock with his fist as he passed it. He ran past the principal's office, out the school's front doors, and onto the playground. He did not seem to know what had propelled him outside, and he didn't know where to go next, but he kept moving. The principal, alerted by Alex's teacher and the sound of breaking glass, ran after him, and ordered him back inside. Alex ignored the principal and kept running, across a grassy soccer field and toward a small, pebbly creek that bordered the school grounds. The principal followed and pleaded with Alex to come back, but Alex kept moving. Worried that Alex might hurt himself or disappear into the neighborhood beyond the creek, the principal ran back to his office and called my wife, Liz, who worked nearby. The only alternative, the principal said, was to call the police.

Liz left work and drove to the school. When she arrived, two policemen were there, trying to coax Alex into a squad car. He wouldn't let them get near him. He stood on the soccer field, frozen, waiting for their next move. When they tried to corner him, he fled. A second police car arrived. Three policemen ran after Alex through backyards and between houses, hopping over fences, scrambling to surround him. Alex grabbed a fallen tree limb and swung it at the officers as they approached. They briefly retreated, but he couldn't keep them all away. Moments later, they got close enough to grab him. Alex was screaming, punching, and kicking. Two of the policemen wrestled him to the ground, held him, muscled him into the squad car, and locked the doors. As they drove away, he banged his head and kicked his feet against the inside of the car. Liz could hear his muted cries for help.

The police took Alex to the emergency room at the local hospital around noon. The hospital did not have a psychiatric unit, so the staff began arranging for a transfer to a children's psychiatric hospital. Liz called me. I was at my office in Manhattan, where I worked as an editor at *BusinessWeek* magazine. I left the office as soon as I got her call. It was an agonizing two-hour trip on the commuter train from the office to my home, in Ridgewood, a suburb in northern New Jersey. I had no cell phone, no way of keeping in touch, no way of knowing what might be happening. I had only scattered details; Alex had been subdued by the police, locked inside a police car, and taken to the hospital. Did that mean he was under arrest? What had he done? I wished I had stayed on the phone longer before running for the train.

When I got to the emergency room, Alex was lying quietly in a hospital bed, barely able to raise his head. He had fallen asleep shortly after he arrived. He was drained, empty of all the anger, empty of any feeling at all. He looked up at me drowsily. I asked him why he had run out of school. He didn't know. He said he couldn't remember any of the morning's events. He was as confused about what was going on as the rest of us. It seemed the crisis was past. The eleven-year-old who had been strong enough to fight off three policemen a few hours earlier was now a sleepy little boy, worried about what might be coming next.

The doctors in the emergency room said Alex belonged in the county psychiatric hospital. All I knew about the county hospital was that it had recently been the subject of newspaper articles reporting an unusually high incidence of suicide among its adolescent patients. Liz and I scrambled to find an alternative. It took hours to find one and to arrange an ambulance for the trip. Night had fallen by the time the ambulance arrived. I watched as Alex, now calm and still sleepy, was picked up and laid on the gurney. The ambulance driver and his partner chatted pleasantly with Alex as they cinched leather straps around his wrists and ankles. One was a competitive roller skater, who, as he was sliding the gurney into the back of the ambulance, told Alex that he skated not on in-line skates, like the ones Alex had, but on old-fashioned four-wheel skates, or "quads." Then the skater climbed in and closed the door.

In the car now, following that ambulance, I am trying to

focus on my driving, but I'm overwhelmed by doubt and confusion. Why is Alex being treated like a prisoner? I should be taking him home, not driving through the dark to some rural New Jersey town I've never heard of, to a hospital I've never seen, where I am supposed to leave him in the custody of strangers. Boonton Township, the community is called. I begin to worry about money. I work long hours, and I write books and magazine articles on the side, because, despite the long hours, my salary doesn't cover the family's expenses. I haven't been able to set aside money for emergencies, and I can't afford medical bills. When I remember Alex, strapped inside the ambulance in front of me, I am ashamed that I'm thinking about myself. I wonder how his small frame held all that anger. I don't know what to do. I feel frightened and alone as I drive on in blackness broken only by the occasional flash of a passing car's headlights.

Alex is wheeled into the admissions area, where I am handed a stack of forms to fill out. The ambulance attendants chat with Alex as they remove his belt and shoelaces. For a moment I don't understand, and then I do. They think Alex might kill himself. They unstrap him, and he gets up to walk with Liz and me, and someone from the hospital, to the place where he will be staying. We walk down a long hallway, with tile floors and pale yellow cinder-block walls. The woman from the hospital unlocks a door, and we enter a large recreation room. Two dozen children, most of them older than Alex, are playing, relaxing, and joking. It's noisy, but no noisier than an art or physical education class at Alex's school. Who are these children? They look normal. A few seem a little rambunctious, but I wouldn't know they were mentally ill. If that is what they are. One girl sits alone in a chair. I wonder why she is here. I look at other children and wonder the same thing. They seem normal enough to me, but what had I expected? I'd never seen a kid with mental illness. This must be what they look like. Just like other kids. I suppose I had been hoping they would look sick, or different somehow from Alex, so I would know he was not one of them.

After a few minutes, a woman from the hospital tells Liz and me it is time to say good night. I don't see how I can leave. That's my son, and he doesn't know anyone here. The woman is understanding, but firm. Alex is taking this better than I am. He hugs me and hugs his mother and starts to look around the room, trying to find an opportunity to join in. Liz and I walk out the door. I look back at Alex through the small cross-hatched window of reinforced glass in the door. I see him. A hospital staffer puts her hands on Alex's shoulders and walks him out of view. Standing in the empty hallway, I hear the cold, metallic clang of a bolt as the door is locked. It echoes from the tile floor and cinder-block walls. It is the most forlorn sound I have ever heard. Liz and I walk separately, back toward the hospital entrance, not speaking. I'm crying, and I'm embarrassed. I don't look at her. Alex is alone on the other side of that locked door, without me, and I do not have a key.

All I could think of in the days that followed was getting Alex home, getting him better. I wanted this problem fixed. I wanted Alex back in school, and I wanted to forget this horrible thing. I didn't want to write down what happened. I didn't want to think about any of it again, ever. We were having a bad week. I was sure it would soon be over, and we would move on.

I was wrong. That cold night marked the beginning of the saddest and most difficult years of my life. Four years after

Alex was first hospitalized, his younger sister, Alicia, was also admitted to a psychiatric hospital. She was then twelve and in the seventh grade. It had taken years to get Alex a proper diagnosis, and longer to find appropriate treatment. Now we would have to begin again with Alicia.

The oldest of our three children, Matt, responded to all of this by working even harder in school, by keeping to a strict schedule, and by staying late for track practice, his work on the high school paper, and other extracurriculars. He was doing his best to create some order in his life.

In the early years of Alex's and Alicia's illnesses, Liz and I made bad decisions about their care. We didn't understand their illnesses, and we didn't know what to do to help them. I have never suffered from depression, nor have I seen it in my family, or in anyone close to me. I know what it is like to be sad and lonely, and I made the mistake of thinking that depression was like that, only worse. I'd always been able to shake off feelings of sadness and despair, and I thought my kids could too. What they needed to climb out of that state of mind, I was convinced, was simply the will to do it. If my children couldn't summon the strength to cheer themselves up and get on with their lives, I was going to help them do it, or make them do it. We will pull together, I thought. We will get through this.

As a reporter, I had access to the nation's leading psychiatrists and researchers, and I knew where to go for information on psychiatric illnesses in children. But I didn't use any of those resources. I didn't make any calls. I didn't search the medical journals, or browse in bookstores. Why? I'm not entirely sure, but part of the reason was that I was deeply skeptical of psychiatrists and their medications. I was not eager to put my kids in their care. Another reason was that I didn't think it was right to take advantage of my professional contacts to solve my personal problems. But mostly it was because I couldn't admit to myself that my children were in serious trouble. This will be over soon, I thought. Nobody in my family is going to succumb to depression, or anything else. I will not let it happen. *We will get through this.*

As the troubles at home continued, my job as a writer and editor in New York became my refuge. At work, I was successful. I was praised for what I did, and my colleagues thought well of me. At home, nothing seemed to turn out right. No matter what I did, no matter how much effort I expended, things were not getting better. Every evening, as I walked home from the train station, my mood would sink as I neared the house. All I could think about was what fresh crisis might be waiting for me. I felt like a failure as a father, and, increasingly, I couldn't tolerate that feeling.

It took me a long time to learn that I could not solve these problems myself, could not make the children's problems go away. Asking a depressed child to shake off depression is like asking a cancer patient to shake off a tumor. It doesn't work. I thought my children needed tough love, but toughness made them feel as though they were responsible for their illnesses. They were turning against me.

We needed help from someone. But when we tried to find it, it wasn't there. We took the children to a series of psychiatrists who repeatedly misdiagnosed them and treated them incorrectly, sometimes making them worse. We talked to therapists who threw us off course again and again with faulty assessments. We took the children to hospitals that did not keep them long enough to help them, because our insurance company wouldn't pay for the care. We talked to school officials who must have seen dozens or hundreds of troubled kids, but who told us they'd never seen such problems before and had no idea what to do. We spent tens of thousands of dollars, some of the money wasted on inappropriate care, to try to fill the vast gaps in our insurance plan. Sometimes these efforts helped, sometimes they didn't.

What we found was a splintered, chaotic mental health care system that seemed to do more harm than good.

We were not alone. We did not know it then, but an estimated 20 percent of American children and adolescents, or about 15 million of them, experience a diagnosable mental illness in the course of a year, according to the U.S. Surgeon General. Some 6 million to 9 million of those children and adolescents have serious emotional disturbances that can have a significant impact on their lives. These include anxiety disorders, attention-deficit/hyperactivity disorder, depression, bipolar disorder, eating disorders, schizophrenia, Tourette's syndrome, autism, and Asperger's syndrome. Some of these children are so ill they are barely able to function. About three fourths of them fail to receive mental health care, and most receive no health care at all.

Before my children got sick, I'd heard statistics like these, but I didn't believe them. If mental illness was so common in children, why didn't I know any mentally ill kids? I suspected a conspiracy: well-intentioned children's advocates were inflating the statistics to attract support for the cause.

My suspicions dissolved when, several years after Alex's first hospitalization, I began to talk about my children to friends and colleagues. When they asked what I was working on, I would tell them it was a memoir of my experiences with my children's depression. Many of them responded with a story about a nephew, a brother or sister, a cousin, or one of their own children. People I'd known for years would blurt out things they hadn't told anyone, once they knew about my experience.

The statistics about the prevalence of mental illness in children are correct. But it's a hidden epidemic. Millions of families are alone in coping with the ordeal of children's mental illness, unaware of how many others are struggling, too. We all know what it means to sit alone, at night, with a child who might at any moment take a swing at us or another of our children, or run out the back door, or grab a kitchen knife, or swallow a bottle of pills. We know what it's like to send a child away, to surrender the care of our children to strangers, and to have medical decisions made by anonymous insurance executives. Too many families know what it's like to lose a child, because they couldn't find help in time. Children and adolescents with mental illness are among the most neglected and mistreated members of our society.

The epidemic of mental illness in children is all around us, but it's not something we talk about easily. I didn't. In the days after Alex was admitted to the hospital, I told people that he had a bad case of the flu. "Don't tell anyone at school what's happening," I told Liz. "We don't want the other parents to be afraid to let their kids play with Alex."

My attitude has completely changed since then. I now know that it's crucial that we talk about it. The longer the epidemic remains hidden, the longer it will continue.

Alex and Alicia agreed to let me tell their stories. I've examined more than a thousand pages of their medical records. We have spent many hours in therapy together. And I interviewed them, to give them an opportunity to include their views in this story, especially when those views differ from mine. Alicia allowed me to look through a remarkable series of journals she kept during the worst years of her illness.

Matt was opposed to this project. He was concerned about the way I would portray Alex, Alicia, and Liz. He agreed to be interviewed, but only so he could add what he thought were crucial details. His interpretation of events was often quite different from mine, and he didn't want his participation to be construed as an endorsement of the book. He asked me not to quote him, except in instances in which he gave me explicit permission to do so.

I've told this story exactly as I remember it, checking dates and details wherever possible against medical and insurance records. The only thing I have changed is the names and some of the identifying characteristics of children other than my own.

CHAPTER ONE

t is the spring of 1996, after Alex's first hospitalization. He is eleven years old and in the fifth grade. He has left the hospital with no diagnosis. No one has told us what treatment he needs, or how we should proceed. He and his teacher, with whom he'd begun the year in an uneasy stand-off, are now openly at war. It was Alex's sometimes rambunctious behavior in class, talking out of turn and cracking jokes at the wrong times, that had initially put her on her guard. But his explosive emotional outbursts, which now occur once or twice a week, have long since depleted her patience. Despite the hospitalization, the examinations, and the tests, we have no idea what is causing these emotional storms. Neither does Alex, who is as puzzled by his behavior as we are. His teacher isn't puzzled, however. She thinks she knows exactly what is going on: Alex is bent on attacking her, and all this talk about psychiatric problems is nonsense. He is a bad kid, who time and again has interfered with what she is trying to accomplish in class. She wants him out of there, but it is a small school, with only one fifth-grade class, and there is nowhere for him to go. She makes no secret of her distaste. Alex sees it as clearly as we do.

The outbursts are becoming more common at home,

too. Liz and I know that he needs help, that the hospitalization was a failure, but we have no idea what to do. I am inclined to respond with ever stiffer punishment. We might not understand what is going on inside him, but if we're tough, we can control this behavior. Sometimes Liz agrees, and sometimes she doesn't. I can't pin her down on a plan of action. We argue about it often.

One quiet Sunday afternoon at home, some trivial incident I've forgotten prompts an outburst. Alex is screaming, thrashing around the house, gripped by a boiling anger. I know immediately that it will be a long, difficult afternoon and evening before he settles down. He flings open the back door, runs out of the house and down the street to where it ends at railroad tracks. I run after him. He keeps going, through a thicket of weeds and scruffy saplings, down a small embankment and onto the crumbled, gray rocks beside the tracks. At the embankment I look in both directions, to where the tracks, shiny and polished from frequent use, wink out of sight in the distance. There are no trains in view now, but this is a busy line, shared by New York City commuter trains and freights. Alex is crouching on the rocks, not far from the tracks. "I'm going to stand in front of the train and die," he screams. He waits. I stand near the trees, where he can see me. I dare not move closer, for fear he will run onto the tracks. I try to coax him toward me. He turns away and looks at the tracks. I wait. He picks up a rock and tosses it toward the rails. A faint breeze stirs the trees. I have no idea whether he is serious about jumping in front of a train. Is this a cry for help, or does he really mean to die? After a few long minutes, I ask him to come back to the house and talk. He doesn't say anything. I am growing frantic, wondering whether I should run down and grab him and drag him away from the tracks, but I'm not sure I can catch him. I'm not sure of anything, except that I'm ready to explode. These could be the last minutes I see Alex alive.

Liz is behind me; I don't know exactly where. I don't expect any help from her. We never agree on what to do about Alex, even in calm moments. We certainly won't be able to work out a plan now. I watch Alex and try to edge closer, but he moves away, closer to the tracks. Trembling, I stumble backward through the trees, back to the house, leaving Alex there alone. I need to call someone. But whom? An ambulance? The psychiatrist Alex has seen twice? It is a Sunday; the psychiatrist's office is closed, and there is no answering service or night number. This guy doesn't do emergencies. In desperation, I call the police. "My son is sitting by the railroad tracks, threatening to kill himself," I say with a shaking voice. "Can you come and get him?" They will send a car over, an officer tells me. I put down the phone and jog back to the tracks, to keep an eye on Alex. I wonder what the police will do. He isn't threatening anyone but himself. Can they arrest him? And I wonder what kind of father I've become, turning over the care of my child to a stranger in a blue uniform.

A police car arrives a few minutes later, quietly, with no lights flashing and no siren. I move away, where I can watch but stay out of the patrolman's way. He walks up to Alex, saying something I can't hear. Alex follows him to the police car and gets into the backseat. The policeman calls to me. "Follow me to the station in a few minutes," he says. He gets into the car and drives away with Alex.

Liz and I silently get into the car and drive to the station, leaving Matt, fourteen, and Alicia, nine, at home. We are brought into a small, bare room, with a couple of scarred, dark green metal desks and a few chairs, where a police officer has been talking to Alex. I can't tell whether this is the officer who took him away; my mind is too fogged to be able to tell one from another. I don't know what he has said, but Alex seems a little better now. He meets my eye briefly, uneasily, before looking away again. We talk with the policeman and Alex for an hour or two about what has been bothering Alex and what he might do to calm himself. Then we take Alex home. We wait. We try to eat. We watch him. We move slowly around the house. Nobody talks much. We don't know how to keep this from happening again.

It's difficult to say where this story begins. Alex was a happy, bright-eyed child. He loved roughhousing and was always nicking a shin or twisting an ankle. He was friendly and affectionate, and liked to play with his older brother. For the first few years of Alex's life, Matt and Alex were best friends. Alex wasn't happy being alone. He was always looking for playmates, and he made friends easily. He could be shy with adults, but he was comfortable with other kids. From the time he was a toddler, he was taller and stronger than most other children his age, but he was far too gentle to use his size or strength to bully anyone. He was funny; he would win over the other kids by making them laugh. When he was excited, he'd be charged with nervous energy, bouncing one leg up and down when sitting in a chair, fidgeting, and absentmindedly twirling his blond curls around his finger.

Along with his size came a precocious athletic ability. I was one of those kids who, during pickup baseball games, is always chosen last and parked in right field, the traditional refuge of those who can neither catch the ball nor throw it very well. Alex, on the other hand, was a natural athlete. I was amazed by what he could do. He knew how to catch and throw a baseball from the first time he picked one up. All he wanted to do was play catch, or hockey, or basketball, or football. What he lacked as an athlete was competitiveness and aggressiveness. He was too gentle and amiable to want to vanquish an opponent.

He seemed to have a special talent for baseball, and he looked like a ballplayer. On the field, he assumed just the right slouch between plays (how do kids learn that?), but he sprang into readiness, punching his mitt and bending his knees, whenever a batter stepped up to the plate. Because he was good, when he started Little League he was asked if he'd like to pitch. I encouraged him to give it a try; he had a strong delivery, and I thought he would excel as a pitcher. He pitched one or two innings, over the course of several games, and then lost any interest: though he pitched well, he was overwhelmed by the pressure of being alone on the mound, with all eyes on him and the game depending heavily on his performance. When he gave up a hit or a run, he'd come back to the bench in tears. He didn't want to be a pitcher, he told me. I ached to see him so upset, and I worried, a little, that I'd pushed him too hard. But I'd encouraged him only because he was good at it, and he liked it. I was sorry to see baseball make him sad.

Alex was a natural builder. If I left a few pieces of scrap wood on the floor in my basement workshop, Alex would disappear down there. After an hour or two of banging, cutting, and sanding, he'd emerge and ask me to drill a couple of holes for him. The projects varied, from a table for his room to a shelf for his model cars. For one school project, he designed an alarm system for his room, so he would know when his brother was coming. I wondered whether he might become an engineer or an architect one day.

Alex was easily the most injury-prone of the three kids. When he was two years old, he and Liz were coming out of a Chinese restaurant with a bag of takeout food when Alex tripped on the sidewalk, fell, and hit his head. He might have been unconscious for a moment; she couldn't tell. Somebody called an ambulance, and he was taken to the emergency room. As far as doctors could determine, the fall did no damage. That was the first of what would be a dozen or so trips to emergency rooms. Alex broke his wrist twice, one of his feet, an arm, and I'm not sure what else. That's not counting the pulls, tears, twists, and bruises that seemed serious but turned out not to be.

Alex's most serious injury occurred when he was six. We were on a family vacation with my parents in northern Michigan, when I stopped the car on a causeway to take a picture of a sunset over the water. I walked across the road and was standing on the opposite shoulder, focusing my camera, when Alex jumped out of the car and ran toward me. He didn't look for traffic. "Daddy!" he yelled, with his arms stretched out toward me and a big smile on his face. I turned just in time to see the smile replaced by a confused, wide-eyed look as he was scooped up by the front bumper of an oncoming car. The collision threw him up onto the hood of the car, near the windshield. As the car slowed and stopped, he rolled forward, tumbling off the car and onto the ground. I ran toward him, howling with anger and disbelief. There was no other traffic on the road; only my car, and the car that had hit him. He landed on his face and was rolling over onto his back as I got to him. He was conscious, and slightly stunned. He wasn't crying. We were miles from a hospital, a doctor, or even a telephone. Knowing that it was wrong to pick up someone who was injured, for fear of aggravating the injuries, I picked him up anyway, and put him in the backseat with Liz.

By this time, a passing car had stopped. The driver said there was a doctor about ten miles away, and he gave me quick directions. Behind the wheel of the car that hit Alex sat an elderly woman, alone. She stared straight ahead, with her hands covering her mouth. She didn't move. When she hit Alex, she had been driving below the speed limit, perhaps only twenty or twenty-five miles an hour. If she'd been going any faster, Alex probably would have been killed.

I sped off with Alex in the back. He was now crying, and yelling, "It hurts! It hurts!" We got to the doctor's office, where in my confusion, I waited in line behind a patient talking to the receptionist through a window. Liz ran in and shouted, "We have a boy who was hit by a car. It's an emergency." The doctor ran outside with a stretcher, brought Alex inside, examined him, and determined that he should be moved to a hospital. An ambulance arrived a few minutes later; I rode in the front, Liz rode with Alex in the back, and my parents followed in our car, with Matt and Alicia. During the forty-five-minute ride, I overheard one of the emergency medical technicians radio the hospital, saying "Patient's left eye is dilated." I didn't know exactly what that meant, but I knew it wasn't good. At the hospital, after a series of CT scans and physical exams, the doctors said that Alex, miraculously, had suffered only a broken leg. His mental faculties seemed fine; the ambulance technician had been mistaken about the dilation of the eye. Could the accident have caused some subtle brain damage that wasn't apparent at the time? Nothing turned up in any of the tests, so the answer is probably not. But it's impossible to be sure.

The only hint of the emotional troubles Alex would experience later came when he was four years old and in nursery school. One of his teachers called Liz and me to the school for a conference. She said she was concerned about the way Alex was behaving with his classmates. It was something about the way he played with the other children; he wasn't connecting with them as he should be. Perhaps, she said, we should have him evaluated by a therapist. We thanked her and left, before I had a chance to blurt out what I was thinking: You must be out of your mind. A four-year-old seeing a therapist? Don't tell me my child needs a therapist. Maybe you're the one who needs an evaluation.

In first grade, Alex was a bright and eager student. A few months into the school year, his teacher wrote on his report card that he was capable of working independently, enjoyed participating in group discussions, enjoyed writing, and took pride in his written work. He was a good reader, and he pushed himself to take on more difficult books. The only troubling points on his first report card were that he was sluggish in the morning and that he sometimes got sidetracked during class and had to complete his assignments during recess. He continued to advance the following year. "Alex has grown into quite a writer," his second-grade teacher wrote. He began to display a particular talent for math and for research, or what passes for research in the second grade: "Alex has a very inventive mind and is filled with interesting insights." He was soon asking for extra math assignments, and he represented his class in a school-wide mathematics competition. He was becoming a leader in class discussions and projects. There were times, his teacher noted, when he was easily distracted by others and his behavior was "inappropriate." He'd make a wisecrack that disrupted the class, or joke with other students during group projects. These "obstacles" sometimes interfered with his development "as an independent learner." Even so, she concluded that he was "a very capable student with mature interests and learning goals." At the end of the school year, Alex's good reports were tempered with similar concerns. "Our goal continues to be appropriateness in his behavior," his teacher wrote. "He realizes that he can work much more efficiently when he has self-control."

The teachers didn't emphasize these concerns in our meetings with them, presumably because Alex was doing so well. I don't remember asking about his "inappropriate behavior." I might have been able to do something at home to help Alex develop more self-control—or, more likely, it would have become an issue over which Liz and I argued. We had, by then, a long history of arguing over the children. When we encountered a problem with the kids' behavior, I usually took a tougher stance than she did. We can't allow this, I would say. If they get away with it now, what happens when they are teenagers? How will we maintain any control over them?

You're too hard on them, she would reply. Leave them alone. And besides, I don't care what you think; I'm not going to enforce your rules when you're at work or away. We never found a way to resolve these disputes. Neither of us could stick with the compromises we sometimes reached. In the case of Alex's "inappropriate behavior," we didn't do anything. It didn't seem like a big problem. I was pleased with Alex's overall growth and development, and I thought perhaps his teacher was being a little too scrupulous in her demands. Alex was a rough-and-tumble kid. If he misbehaved a little in class, that was a small concern, especially when compared with his accomplishments.

During the next couple of years, Alex continued to do well in school. He played soccer until he was old enough to join Little League and play baseball. He and Matt spent less time together as they got older, and each developed a separate set of friends at school. They began to spar in the way that brothers often do, but their clashes were short-lived and they continued to get along well.

By the fourth grade, though, Alex's teachers were displaying more concern. The child who had excelled in math two years earlier was now making careless mistakes. He'd lost some of his enthusiasm for writing, but was still "capable of completing reflective pieces." Given writing assignments, Alex often wrote about what was evidently his favorite subject—his car accident. Sometimes he illustrated these papers with a crayon drawing of himself being struck and thrown on the road. Whenever I asked him what he thought about the accident, he would repeat what he'd put into his compositions, which mostly just retold the story. Were we missing something? He seemed fixated on the episode, but it was hard to know why. Maybe there had been some emotional aftereffects; or maybe he liked to retell the story because he was the hero, the superman who had survived what could easily have been a fatal accident. Perhaps we should have made more of this fascination and taken Alex to see someone who could help sort out what was going on. But we didn't.

In the spring of fourth grade, Alex's teacher asked Liz and me to meet with her one morning before school started, to talk about Alex's behavior in the classroom. I called the office to say I'd be late, and we drove the four blocks to the school, with Alex. The teacher was sitting at her desk in the classroom when we arrived. It was uncomfortably warm; sunlight poured through the venetian blinds. The room smelled of musty books and chalk. Alex sat down, and Liz and the teacher and I wedged into students' desks as the teacher explained that Alex was becoming increasingly disruptive in class, making it difficult for the other children to do their work. Sometimes he would work happily for a while, then darken and turn angry. He would speak out of turn; he'd make cracks about assignments and announce that he wasn't going to do them. The swagger was intended to impress the other kids, or make them laugh, I figured. This wasn't so serious. I didn't know why he'd decided this was the way he was going to earn his stripes among his peers, but I wasn't too concerned. Maybe the teacher was missing something in the classroom. Maybe the other kids were putting Alex up to it, or maybe he was frustrated by the work or reacting too strongly to the teacher's rebukes.

None of this worried me. What did worry me was the way Alex reacted to the criticism that morning. He listened until he'd heard enough, then stood abruptly and walked toward the far corner of the room, near the louvered windows, pretending not to listen, looking out from under his light brown curls with hooded, angry eyes. Instantly infuriated by this show of disrespect to his teacher and his parents, I followed him and sputtered, in an angry stage whisper, "You get back into your seat and listen to your teacher. Now." He refused. The angry defiance in his eyes was something I'd never seen before. With the teacher watching, I fought the impulse to shout, or to grab him by the arm and muscle him back to his desk. I leaned into his face and in a coarse whisper said again, "Get back there now." By this time I'd lost track of what the teacher had been saying, because I was so outraged by the show of disrespect.

Alex didn't move. In the standoff, I thought briefly of my father, of how I would never have dared to treat him this way. Powerless, I left Alex standing in the corner. He remained by the windows while the rest of us finished the conversation without him. Later, on the train to New York, I was still angry with him, but I also felt a certain grudging admiration. He's a tough kid, I thought. At the age of ten, he'd had the fortitude to resist the combined authority of his parents and his teacher. When I was his age, a sharp look would leave me quivering. It seemed clear that it was time to teach Alex some respect. If he was refusing to listen to his teacher and his parents at ten, how would he behave at sixteen? Best to step in right away, I reasoned, to be stern with him at home and to encourage his teacher to do the same, until he learned that this behavior would not be tolerated. It seemed harsh, but I didn't know what else to do. I thought about the scattered reports, in earlier grades, that Alex's behavior had been inappropriate, and I wondered whether there might be more to all of this than I had presumed. The message in those reports was starting to worry me a little, but I continued to believe that the problem would resolve itself as he got older.

He got through the remaining months of fourth grade with occasional rebukes from his teacher, but nothing serious enough to require another special parent-teacher conference. I never did deliver the tough response that I thought his behavior deserved. I didn't want to be the bad guy, and anyway he seemed to be doing better. It was easy to believe that the problem had disappeared. He spent the summer as he always did, constantly out of the house, playing with the neighborhood kids. He went to summer camp for two weeks, and came back bubbling with enthusiasm over the experience. Away from school, in the warm months of summer, whatever disciplinary problems he was having melted away.

In September, when Alex started fifth grade, the problems with classroom behavior resumed, and now they were more serious. Alex was one of the oldest kids in the fifth grade—he had just missed the age cutoff for starting kindergarten—and most of his friends had been in the grade ahead of his. They had now moved on to middle school, and while that didn't preclude playing together, the unwritten social rules dictated that middle school kids shouldn't be seen hanging out with kids from the elementary school. He was adrift, socially.

Only a few weeks into the year, he began to fall behind in his work. He missed school frequently. After I had left for work, he would claim to be suffering from one affliction or another, and Liz usually let him stay home. When he was in school, he was regularly sent to the principal's office for disrupting class. Alex and the other fifth-graders were in an experimental project in which two classes, each with about twenty-five students, had been combined in one large room, with joint supervision by two teachers. The idea was to create a more open classroom, in which students could move from one study area to another, working independently and on group projects. It was an interesting idea, and it might have worked well for some of the students, but the relative lack of discipline and the freedom to wander were more than Alex could handle. By the middle of the year, when he was supposed to have read four books, he'd read only one. The trips to the principal's office became more frequent.

This principal was a legendary disciplinarian who had been running the place since it was built, twenty-five years earlier. At first, Alex was afraid of him, as were most of the children and many of their parents. But Alex's fear soon dissipated, and he began to relish dismissals from the classroom. When instructed to go to the principal's office, he'd roam through the school instead. He would boast to the other kids that he hadn't gone, shrugging off the possibility of even more severe punishment. The other children admired him, and feared him a little, too.

We were getting desperate. The principal thought Alex might benefit from a little therapy. I was instantly on my guard. I didn't like the idea that he would have to face someone alone. The school was probably partly responsible for what was happening with him, and so were Liz and I. Whatever was going on, it didn't seem as though all the blame should be placed on Alex. And that's what I thought would happen if he saw a therapist. I didn't say that to the principal—I didn't say anything; I didn't want to give him the opportunity to try to change my mind. But, later, I thought about the recommendation. Maybe therapy wouldn't be so bad for Alex. There was even a chance he would find it helpful. And, in any case, it would get the principal off my back. We found a psychologist in town who saw children Alex's age, and Alex went to see him four or five times. It was a disaster. Alex fought when it was time to go; sometimes the promise of a trip to McDonald's afterward would help get him to his appointments, and sometimes it wouldn't. When we could get him to the office, he argued and shouted during the entire session, demanding to know why he was there and what he was being blamed for. He said the therapist was stupid, didn't know anything, and couldn't help. We gave up. Alex was relieved, and so, I suspect, was the therapist.

At school, it was not only the other students who were

afraid of Alex; his teacher was afraid of him, too. She didn't know how to control him, and when she asked for advice, Liz and I didn't know what to tell her. The same things were happening at home. He wouldn't listen to his mother or to me. He wouldn't come to the table when dinner was ready, he wouldn't come into the house when he was told to, and he stopped doing homework. He began wearing a red bandanna as a do-rag, wrapped tightly across his forehead and tied at the back of his neck. It was a tough, defiant look, and to anyone who didn't know that a gentle soul was concealed under that swagger, it was intimidating.

It seemed clear that Alex was trying to frighten the kids and the teacher, but why? When Alex wasn't sparring with the teacher, getting booted from class, or confronting the principal, he was smiling and joking with the other kids. His laughter and good nature belied his tough appearance, except when the calm gave way to an emotional storm. Whatever effect the outbursts were having on the students and teachers at school, they were having a much more serious effect on him. He looked far too worn and tired for a healthy eleven-year-old.

His teacher showed little compassion. She might have approached Alex with some understanding that he was in a difficult emotional place, even while doing what she had to do to maintain a proper atmosphere in her classroom. Instead, she treated him like an incipient criminal. He was a bad kid, she told the principal, and she wanted him out of her class. That might have been good for both of them, but there was nowhere for Alex to go. All fifty of the school's fifth-graders were in the same experimental program, under her direction.

So she did what she could to make his life as unpleasant

as possible, perhaps hoping that he would stay home more often. Along with his classmates, he had been rehearsing for several weeks for the spring vocal concert. A week before the performance, she dismissed him from the chorus. He told us he didn't care about that concert anyway, but he was hurt. I understood the teacher's concern; Alex had been disrupting rehearsals. But it was almost time for the concert, and surely she could have endured one more week with him. Dismissal seemed too severe a punishment. I was disappointed for him. He had been looking forward to the concert, and I had, too.

I wanted to do something for him, but there was nothing to do. In the days before the concert, his emotional state deteriorated until he was almost unable to function. He missed several days of school. The night of the concert, he said he felt better, even though he'd missed that day at school, and he said he wanted to attend the performance. I took him to the concert, in the school gym, where parents were gathering in folding chairs. He put on the red bandanna and took a seat away from me, alone, in the middle of the audience. I sat near the back, watching. I was surprised that he'd wanted to go, considering his disappointment over being dismissed from the show. He was quiet, listened respectfully to the music, and joked with his friends afterward. I was proud of him for going, but his teacher saw it differently. She was convinced he was there to intimidate the kids who were singing. Later, she claimed that she could see him giving each one of them a threatening look.

All of this had happened before anyone suggested that Alex might be suffering from an emotional disorder, and I blamed Alex's teacher for most of the problems. He could be a difficult kid, sure, but most eleven-year-olds had their difficult days. If she hadn't turned against him, I thought, most of this wouldn't have happened. What must it feel like to Alex, to be actively disliked by his teacher, the person who ruled his universe away from home? Yet it was becoming clear to everyone, even to me, that Alex would need more help than Liz or I could give him. The episode by the railroad tracks and the problems in school added up to something I didn't understand.

I still thought the school should do more. But I began to entertain the thought that the school wasn't solely responsible for Alex's troubles. Maybe Liz and I were part of Alex's problem. Maybe we were not very good parents. We loved Alex, and we both tried to do our best. But we weren't very good at working together. We were never able to talk about what was happening with him without pointing fingers at each other. Maybe I'd had too pleasant a childhood to be a good parent. I was raised in a mostly happy home, and I thought I could do at least as good a job as my parents, maybe better. My parents had made it look easy. Now I was starting to doubt my abilities. Maybe this was something I had no talent for. I'd been a parent long enough to know that it was a difficult job that requires patience, empathy, understanding, and emotional endurance, enough to last for eighteen or twenty years. I was sure I had the endurance, but I wasn't so sure about the patience, empathy, and understanding. I was often impatient, and I wasn't a very good listener. I was much more comfortable instructing the kids, telling them what they ought to be thinking or doing, than I was listening to them.

While I was entertaining these doubts, Liz and I were arguing more and more, it seemed. I knew that was a problem, too, but I didn't know how to solve it. At first, I thought that our disagreements, as heated and unpleasant as they often became, were a normal part of marriage; but the relationship we had built and polished for the first five or six years we were together was becoming tarnished. The arguments left hurts that accumulated like barnacles, weighing us down and leaving sharp, exposed edges. But didn't that happen to everyone as the years went by? Most of my friends seemed to be in the same situation. It wasn't unusual at work to see someone clutching a phone and leaning over a desk, trying to muffle an exchange of angry words with his or her spouse. Colleagues who traveled out of town for work, as I did, traded stories about the frosty receptions they got when they returned.

I often blamed Liz for our arguments. I told her that she seemed to be enjoying them, that she seemed to get some satisfaction out of creating chaos. When I was angry, I told her she should stop because the arguments were hurting Alex, as well as Matt and Alicia. The arguments continued. We tried going to a family counselor, who met with the family several times and then decided that what we needed was not family therapy, but marital therapy. So Liz and I started going to see her alone, without the children. The sessions were a failure. After an hour with the therapist, venting all our frustration, irritation, and disappointment with each other, we left angrier than when we walked in. We'd keep yelling on the way out of her office, and we often stood in the parking lot arguing for ten or fifteen minutes before we got in the car. We would arrive home fuming; sometimes we would sit in the garage for a few minutes, with the car off, trying to compose ourselves before going inside to see the kids. I don't think we fooled them.

Around this time, Liz started to drink more heavily than

she had in the past. It had been unusual for us to drink during the week, but now the first thing Liz did when she came home from work was pop the tab on a can of Bud Light, sometimes before she took off her coat. She went up to two beers a night, sometimes more. From time to time, I would notice, when I threw a can into the recycling bag, that it was full of empty beer cans. Meanwhile, Liz's doctor prescribed Paxil for what he thought was mild depression. She never saw a psychiatrist. This diagnosis was made by an internist, the same one I saw, the kind of guy who could get through a fifteen-minute appointment in seven or eight minutes. Liz started to see a therapist, irregularly at first, and then more often.

When the kids were young, I worked two jobs. I had a full-time day job—first as a reporter for the Associated Press, later as an editor and writer for *BusinessWeek*. On nights and weekends, I wrote freelance magazine pieces and a couple of books. My earnings were modest by New York City standards, but enough for us. With the help of the extra income from the books and freelancing, I was able to cover the mortgage, the groceries, and gas and electricity, with enough left over for Montessori school tuition, braces, and an occasional vacation, usually by car. We had one car, not two, and a three-bedroom clapboard house that was too small for a family of five. Unlike many of our neighbors in this wealthy town, we did not go skiing in Colorado or snorkeling in the Virgin Islands during winter school breaks. But Liz wanted to be at home with the children when they were young. She temporarily gave up a career as a fund-raiser for nonprofit groups, and I took satisfaction in earning enough money to enable her to do so. We both thought it was good for the kids.

What neither of us anticipated was that Liz wouldn't be happy at home with the kids all the time. A few years after Matt was born, she took a part-time job, but she was still at home far more than I was. She began to complain that I was gone all the time, and she felt that this entitled her to make all the decisions concerning the children without consulting me. She was the one at home enforcing whatever we decided, she said, so she was going to make sure things were decided her way. If I didn't like it, I could stay home with the kids, and she would get a job.

I disagreed. I worked eight hours a day or longer, and commuted three hours on top of that, to support the family, I pointed out; I wasn't ceding my authority to her. It was ridiculous of her to suggest that I stay home with the kids, I told her. By that time, even my modest reporter's salary was several times what she'd been earning when she stopped working. With three children, there was no serious question of switching roles.

Our arguments escalated when Liz ignored this and began to make decisions without me. For about ten years after Matt, our oldest, was born, we managed, at my insistence, to keep the television off on weeknights. The house was quiet and relaxed. Matt could do his homework in the family room, if he chose to, without the television to distract him. I read to Alex and Alicia, or we played board games. (Matt told me later that he would go to friends' houses to catch the afternoon cartoons.) I joked with friends that keeping the TV off was one of the few things Liz and I had managed to do right. On the weekends, the kids could soak up all the television they liked. We didn't put any limits on them from Friday night through Sunday night.

But now, occasionally, I would come home from work and find the television on. The kids, predictably, would be scattered on the floor, absorbed by it. I was astonished. Liz finally told me she'd been letting the kids watch TV after school for months. I protested, and the kids took the opportunity to rush into the breach between us and win the right to endless TV. Before long, the TV was on all the time. Liz liked this, because it helped keep the kids occupied after school; besides, she'd grown bored with reading and games at night.

Another disagreement emerged over whether we would eat dinner together as a family. I thought we should; Liz didn't think it was important. Like many of my neighbors, I commuted to New York by train. I left the house before the children were awake to make the hour-and-a-half-long trip to the office. I was out of town about one week each month. When I wasn't traveling, I left the office at 4:55 every afternoon to catch the 5:47 train out of Hoboken, so that I'd have time to spend with the kids before they went to bed. That meant I got home about 6:30.

The kids had always eaten by the time I got home. Sometimes Liz waited to have dinner with me, and sometimes she didn't. I asked Liz to give the kids snacks in the afternoon, so we could eat dinner together when I got home. She couldn't, she said; the kids were too hungry, and they couldn't wait. On weekends, if I didn't get to the kitchen first, she would make dinner for the kids, feed them, and then start dinner for the two of us.

Some of my fondest memories of childhood are of sitting around the dinner table with my family every night. My parents worked office jobs doing things they didn't have a passion for. It was a way to support the family. (My father worked part-time at night as a musician; that was his passion.) Two or three nights a week, my mother, a secretary, worked evenings as a temp and missed dinner. On those nights, my father cooked and he and my younger sister and I would eat together. But whenever my mother wasn't working, she was there, too. My parents talked about their day at work. I learned everything I know about office politics from my father. My mother liked to tell stories about her high-school escapades. My father's stories about his years in the military during World War II were among my favorites, as were his tales of traveling with a big band as a young saxophone player. My sister and I would always ask to hear the same stories over and over again. It was a doorway into an adult world we weren't part of yet, and we were fascinated by it.

Liz had grown up differently. She had five brothers and sisters, who were always moving in different directions. They did little together, partly because it was hard to round them all up, and partly because her parents had very different jobs. Her father was a doctor. He got up to play tennis at six A.M., was in the hospital by seven or eight to make his rounds, spent all day at his office, and was frequently on call at night. Liz's mother decided to go to college when the kids were young. She was in class several nights a week, and did homework much of the time when she was home. Then she started teaching English at the local community college. It was rare for the family to sit together at one table. But it never seemed to bother them. They joked about how their father couldn't remember their birthdays and their ages. It was a far more laissez-faire arrangement than what I was used to, and it wasn't what I'd envisioned for my young family. I wanted our family to be like mine.

But that was the end of it. We rarely ate dinner as a family, an unfortunate routine that continued when the kids were teenagers and easily able to wait until I got home. The pattern was set. Liz wanted to get the children's dinner out of the way before she and I sat down to dinner. Eating as a family mattered enormously to me, and not at all to her. We seemed incapable of compromise. I felt disenfranchised within my own family.

Part of the reason I worked two jobs was so that we could afford to live in Ridgewood, an upper-middle-class suburb of about 25,000 people at the northern end of New Jersey. Predominantly Republican, populated mostly by lawyers and Wall Street executives and their families, Ridgewood wasn't a perfect fit. As one of only a few people in town who were not registered Republicans, I disagreed with most of my neighbors about politics.

We lived on the "poor" side of town (poor by Ridgewood standards), among the starter houses that young families bought when they wanted to get a toehold in the suburbs. When we moved in, in the late 1980s, the prices for those houses started around $250,000. We managed to find one for a little less; even so, making the mortgage payments was a struggle. Most of the families who bought the small houses would stay a few years and then move into bigger houses across town, or in a neighborhood called the Heights. Few left Ridgewood. The commute to Wall Street was convenient, and moving to any of the other towns in the area would have been a step down.

Ridgewood has a pleasant redbrick downtown, about six blocks long and three blocks wide. It has a movie theater, a post office, two or three dozen restaurants, and the stores that fit the demographics, including Starbucks, Williams-Sonoma, The Gap, and Laura Ashley. On weekends, the sidewalks are clogged with trim blond housewives pushing strollers and holding the hands of their toddlers. Fathers cruise through town in the "bonus cars" they buy with their year-end Wall Street bonuses, which can amount to hundreds of thousands of dollars. The cars might be Lamborghinis or Ferraris, desirable for the nameplate and the bragging rights. Those who are nostalgic about their younger days buy the cars they ogled as teenagers—classic, mint-condition Mustangs or Corvettes. The cars are restored by someone else, of course; few of the owners have time for that sort of work. High school kids wave to one another through the windows of the Mercedes or the little roadsters that their parents buy them, to get them to and from school. It's not unusual for a seventeen-year-old to be given a new car, wreck it, endure a stern admonition, and to be given a new one. The kids park illegally near the high school, collecting tickets every day until they have a stack; then their parents write a check.

The attraction of Ridgewood, for me and many other residents, was its school system. It is, by reputation, one of the best in New Jersey. Ridgewood High School, with its dark, ivy-covered walls and gabled roof, looks more like an expensive prep school than a public institution. It sprawls across a gracefully shaded hill, overlooking football, soccer, and lacrosse fields. It has an exceedingly low dropout rate, and its top graduates attend Yale, Harvard, the University of Chicago, and other such notable institutions. Ridgewood's real-estate-savvy homeowners praise the school for its enviable track record and the quality of its instruction; also, of course, because having a good school system keeps property values high. In Garrison Keillor's Lake Wobegone, all the women are strong, all the men are good-looking, and all the children are above average. In Ridgewood, above average isn't enough. The children have to be in the ninety-eighth percentile, or they are given tutors and sent to supplementary classes. We moved to Ridgewood so that we could give the children a private-school-style education without paying private-school tuition.

With Alex's problems continuing, Liz and I decided, finally, that we would have to take some action. Whatever was responsible for Alex's problems—the school, the deteriorating situation at home, or both—we knew he needed help. The therapist he'd battled with hadn't helped. Maybe he needed medication. We decided to take him to a psychiatrist.

I called my insurance company and asked for the names of some child psychiatrists on its list of preferred providers. I waited, listening to the tapping of a keyboard through the phone line. There were none within fifty miles, said the anonymous voice on the other end. Ridgewood is about twenty-five miles from New York, which must have more psychiatrists per capita than anywhere else on earth, and yet there was not one child psychiatrist on the insurance company's list. We could see a child psychiatrist who was not on the list and pay $250 an hour, only $30 or $40 of which would be reimbursed; or we could see an adult psychiatrist on the preferred-provider list and have most of the cost covered. The woman on the phone gave me a few names.

I called one and made an appointment. A few days later, Alex, Liz, and I went to the psychiatrist's office, in a small, white house on a busy commercial street. Just inside the front door was a cramped waiting room with a dozen or so chairs, all occupied by quiet, downcast middle-aged men and women. The three of us stood quietly in the corner, trying not to make eye contact with any of the other patients. I wasn't sure what was proper behavior in a psychiatrist's office. I'd never been in one.

After a short wait, the receptionist said the doctor was ready to see Alex. We stood up to go in, but she asked us to stay in the waiting room. The doctor wanted to see Alex alone. Before I could protest, Alex disappeared behind the consulting room door. He came out twenty minutes later. I couldn't read anything in his expression.

The doctor would like to see Alex's parents now, the receptionist said. We spent twenty minutes with him, giving him an abbreviated history of Alex's problems. No, there was no clear history of mental illness in either of our families, we told him. Liz said she thought her grandmother had suffered from depression. But she'd lived in Greece, in sometimes difficult circumstances. Who could tell whether she'd been depressed? The doctor said Alex was suffering from depression. He scribbled a prescription and handed it to us. Get this filled, start him on it tomorrow, and set up another appointment in a week or two, he said. We took the prescription, awkwardly thanked him, and left. We collected Alex, picked our way through the crowded waiting room, and left.

I wanted to feel relief, but I didn't. I had hoped that the visit would produce some sort of insight and give me the sense that we were starting something that would help Alex. But it felt more like a dismissal. I'd barely started to explain what had been happening when the time was up. The prescription was for Mellaril, a fifty-year-old drug originally used to treat schizophrenia. I should have asked the psychiatrist why he preferred that drug to Prozac, or any of the newer antidepressants or antianxiety drugs, but I didn't. I could have looked up Mellaril in the *Physicians' Desk Reference,* the bible of prescription drugs, a copy of which sat on my desk at work, but I didn't. Instead, moving like a sleep-walker, I took the prescription to the drugstore and had it filled.

Looking back, I'm not surprised by what might seem to be a stunning lack of curiosity. I was still in the grip of disbelief, unwilling to admit that Alex was seriously ill. Opening a book to look something up would be opening a door to a world I refused to be part of. I was not going to read about psychiatric drugs and mental illness, because I was not going to be the parent of a mentally ill kid. *We are going to get through this.*

Alex grudgingly started taking the Mellaril. We didn't say much about this to Matt and Alicia. I'm not sure what we could have said. We would not have been able to explain the situation very well, because we didn't understand it ourselves. And why burden them with something that was soon going to be dealt with and forgotten?

Over the next few days, Alex got worse. When he wasn't angrily denouncing his teacher or throwing a tantrum at home, sadness seemed to engulf him. He was tired, listless. Sometimes he didn't seem to have the energy to get angry. Now and then he would begin to cry, and say he felt sad and didn't know why. He said he didn't want to live any longer, and he repeated it often.

Alex saw the psychiatrist again about a week after the first visit. This time he was not so cooperative. He refused to respond to the psychiatrist's questions, except to say that no one could help him. "He talked about wanting to harm himself. He doesn't feel like coming to see a 'shrink' and taking 'stupid pills,'" the psychiatrist wrote in Alex's record. This time, the psychiatrist offered a different diagnosis: adjustment reaction of childhood with mixed features, and intermittent explosive disorder. I might not have used the same words, but I could have come up with that "diagnosis" myself.

I'd always been skeptical of psychiatrists. This had a lot to do with my upbringing. I grew up in a working-class suburb of Detroit, in a neighborhood of new, pumpkin-colored brick houses, laid out in rows like Monopoly houses along a grid of oiled dirt roads, on what had recently been farmland. It was a pleasant enough place, and an industrious one. The young parents who bought those small houses, many of them first-generation Americans, were determined to create a better future for themselves and for their children. The way to accomplish that was to be tough, to keep one's eyes fixed on the goal, and to muster the mental discipline needed to get there. People worked hard, mostly on the deafening assembly lines and in the metal-caged tool shops and stockrooms of the automobile factories that sprawled across the Midwestern landscape. When the men had a chance to work overtime, they took it. That was a good way to bank a few extra bucks, and if you turned down overtime when the boss offered it, he might not offer it again. It helped to cover tuition at the Catholic schools to which many of these mostly Polish-American families sent their children. My mother was one of the few mothers who worked, and she did it for the same reason that everyone else did, to try to get ahead, to save some money for the kids' college tuition. If car sales were up and the plants were at peak production, the overtime could continue for weeks. The men endured it, knowing that there would be lean times, too, or maybe a strike the next time contract talks came up. Nobody was depressed, or manic, or emotionally disturbed—there wasn't time for that.

If any of the people I grew up with suffered from mental illness, it never interfered with work. Psychotherapy, psychiatrists, and psychologists were not for people like them. Therapy and therapists were for the wealthy, who had the time and money to indulge themselves, lying on a couch for hours, talking about their childhoods. The neighborhood was rife, however, with what Alex's psychiatrist might have called "intermittent explosive disorder." Noisy arguments were common. My friends and I could hear them from the backyards or the sidewalks, as we passed by on our bikes. We knew the houses where the arguments were going on nonstop, and we snickered as we passed them, glad we didn't live there.

My attitude didn't change as I got older. I was the first person in my family to go to college, and one of the very few kids in the neighborhood to move out of the state. In Boston, where I went to school, I endured the emotional ups and downs of college life, and of life away from home, without the help of a psychiatrist or counselor. I practiced the self-reliance I'd been taught as a child. I was involved, in a small way, with the antiwar effort during the Vietnam years. I was one body among the hundreds of thousands that gathered regularly on the Boston Common, or at the mall near the Washington Monument, and was committed to George McGovern, the Democratic presidential candidate in 1972. Midway through the campaign, McGovern's vice-presidential choice, Thomas Eagleton, admitted that, yes, he had once been under psychiatric care. Support for Eagleton eroded almost immediately. McGovern, who'd initially said he supported Eagleton "1,000 percent," soon dumped him. Such a man, the consensus seemed to be, could not lead the country: he wasn't stable. The episode made a huge impression on me. I didn't have political ambitions, but I vowed that I would

never see a therapist, because to do so might foreclose opportunities of all kinds. It might ruin my future, as it ruined
Eagleton's. And I would never let that happen to my children,
either.

At school, Alex's situation was becoming increasingly difficult. The principal asked whether we would agree to have
Alex evaluated by the school district's psychologist. I didn't
realize it at first, but this was the beginning of a formal
process that could lead to Alex's official classification as a special education student—eligible for special help, but also
marked as a problem. The school psychologist and several
other school officials assembled in what is called a child-
study team. They spent several hours interviewing Alex,
then observed him in class. They gave him a battery of intelligence and personality tests, including a Rorschach inkblot
test. In his report, the psychologist said he saw no unusual
behavior from Alex in the classroom. During reading time,
Alex sat quietly with the other students, absorbed in a book.
The psychologist also noted that Alex's schoolwork "does
not always reflect his superior-level verbal intelligence." The
intelligence tests revealed that Alex had an above-average
verbal IQ of 122 and an overall score of 114. Alex "has the
capability of attaining very good grades in school, assuming
that he is motivated to do so," the psychologist wrote.

In interviews with the child-study team, Alex "revealed a
good sense of humor," an "ability to relate to others with
good emotional warmth," and an ability to express himself
clearly. But the psychologist found Alex lacking in confidence. "I think I'm stupid," Alex told him. Alex revealed
"strong feelings of inadequacy and weakness," and profound

depression. "He has harbored thoughts of harming himself."
When the psychologist asked what his "magic wish" was,
Alex said he'd like to control his anger, and "to believe in
myself." He said that arguments between Liz and me frightened and upset him. He was worried about his younger sister ("She cries when they quarrel") and frightened of me
("I'm scared when he loses his temper"). He wished his
brother would "be nice, and be my friend."

A psychiatrist affiliated with the school system also met
with Alex, and asked how he was doing. Alex blamed his
angry outbursts on the stress of school, and on teachers who
had falsely accused him of something, or denied him privileges extended to other students. He sometimes thought
about hurting or killing himself, and he said he had tried
once to cut his leg with a stick but hadn't succeeded. Asked
about his family, he said, "I don't want to talk about any of
this." During the conversation, Alex was fidgety. The child-
study team's final report concluded that he had problems,
but that they weren't insurmountable. "The combination of
parental support, professional assistance, and Alex's motivation to improve his situation should allow him to become a
better-adjusted, more self-confident and productive student,"
the report concluded.

It was difficult to reconcile Alex's gradual deterioration
in school with this report. He was bright, capable, and had a
good sense of humor, the experts concluded. I knew all that.
But why, then, was he depressed and suicidal? Why did he
think he was stupid and inadequate? I was disturbed by what
Alex had said about the arguments at home, about me, and
about his brother and sister. And I was frightened by his talk
of suicide. How could the child-study team note those problems and then blithely conclude that he was capable of

becoming a confident and productive student? I had no idea what to make of the report. Liz and I didn't talk about it. I filed it and forgot about it.

After Alex had seen the psychiatrist twice, I was more convinced than ever that I had been right to be skeptical. Aside from prescribing medicines, this guy wasn't doing anything to help Alex. He couldn't make up his mind about the diagnosis, nor could he decide what drugs to prescribe. After the second visit, he decided to taper off the Mellaril and start Alex on Zoloft, an antidepressant. Two different drugs in two visits. I suppose I wouldn't have been second-guessing the psychiatrist if Alex had improved. But he didn't. Within a few days of the second visit, he became even more volatile and explosive.

One evening shortly after that visit, he began shouting that he wanted to be in control, wanted to make his own decisions, and would not take any medication. We sent him upstairs to his room, where he started throwing things. He ran downstairs and outside, grabbing branches on trees and breaking them off as he went by. Liz followed him. He turned and threw a tree limb at her. "I'm happy now!" he shouted. "I'm going to kill everyone." He had a smile on his face. "I'll be dead by morning!" he shouted, as he started up the street. Liz started to cry. "Please come home," she said. "Don't do this to us, to your family."

"I don't have a family," Alex said. "I want to be up in the sky on my own private cloud." Then he paused, and something in him changed. The smile disappeared, and he began to shiver uncontrollably. He walked back toward the house. "Was that really me out there?" he asked. "What happened to me?"

A few days later, on a Sunday evening, I lost control. Liz

had run out to pick up something at the drugstore; Alex, Alicia, Matt, and I were home. We were getting ready to go out for a celebratory dinner. Alex was angry, for no reason I could see. His eyes took on a dark cast, and the now familiar dark crescents appeared underneath them. He was sullen. Alicia and I tiptoed around him, trying not to trigger whatever was building inside him. We got ready to go to dinner, but Alex kept delaying. I walked upstairs and found him in the bathroom with the door open, combing his hair. "It's time to go," I said, irritated. "Let's move." He looked at me with cold eyes and made a profane retort that he knew would provoke me. I was enraged. Don't hit him, I can remember thinking. Don't hit him.

I screamed at Alex and ran into the bathroom. Desperately fighting the urge to hit him, I grabbed him by the shoulders, pushed him back toward the toilet, and shoved him down onto the seat. The toilet bowl cracked, and a jet of water shot across the bathroom floor. I let Alex go and ran down two flights of stairs to the basement to turn off the water. Alicia saw me flying past her down the stairs; terrified, she fled out the back door. Alex followed me down the stairs and ran out of the house himself. I turned off the water, ran to the back door, and followed them. I caught up with Alicia half a block away. She cowered as I came near. By now, I was mostly back in control of myself, and already aching over what I'd just done. The crisis was past, but Alex and Alicia didn't know that. I stopped just before I reached Alicia and pleaded with her to go back to the house while I went after her brother. She dropped her head and slowly headed back home. I ran after Alex, who was by now several blocks away. I caught up with him, but he wouldn't let me get near him. I tried to show him that I was calmer, to convince him that it was okay now, I wasn't angry, he would be safe. But still he wouldn't come to me. I gave up and walked back to the house, hoping he would follow. Or I could call the police, to ask them to find him and pick him up. When I walked in the back door, the water that had erupted in the bathroom had leaked through the floor to the kitchen below. Curtains of water were pouring from the kitchen ceiling on to the floor. Alicia sat nearby, curled in a ball on the couch. The celebratory dinner we'd been planning was for her. The date was March 26, 1996. It was her ninth birthday.

If I could take back one day in my life, that would be it.

CHAPTER TWO

I t was a few days later that Alex exploded in school, smashed the clock in the hall, and ran from the principal. That was the April night I found myself in the car, following an ambulance, on a deserted highway. Alex was admitted to St. Clare's Hospital in Boonton Township, New Jersey, on April 19, 1996. I wasn't easily able to accept what had happened. One day, Alex was a kid having trouble in school. The next, he was a patient in a locked hospital ward. It had happened too fast. Before I could adjust to the idea that Alex might need to be hospitalized, he was already there.

At the hospital, as Alex lay on a gurney beside the open door of the cramped admissions office, I fumbled with the admission forms. I was ill-at-ease, and clumsy. I wanted to ask what would happen next, I wanted to meet the doctors, I wanted to know what they would do, how long it would take for Alex to get better, and when he could come home. But I couldn't get any of those questions out. I couldn't think clearly. It took all the concentration I had to fill out the forms and answer the insurance questions. On the long drive home that night, I hunched over the steering wheel. The highway in front of me softened to a watery blur. I wiped away the tears. Liz and I did not speak.

Later, I made notes for a poem I have never completed. I wanted to write something about being battered by powerful winds—the "winds of hell," I wrote melodramatically in my hasty notes. I imagined myself standing on barren ground, with all the trees blown away, so there was no shelter. I leaned into the wind, fighting to remain upright. Next to me, I saw an eleven-year-old boy, also fighting to stand upright, but because he was smaller and lighter, he was nearly being carried off. He looked up at me. I wanted to help him, to keep him from flying away, but I couldn't reach him. I could see the fear and uncertainty in his eyes. Help me, he seemed to be saying. You're my father. Hold on to me. Hold on.

Alex had been admitted on a Friday, not a good time to enter a psychiatric hospital, as I found out. Except in an emergency, psychiatrists and other therapists see patients mostly on weekdays. It would be two days before we would find out much about his condition. At least the hospital kept him safe over the weekend, something I wasn't sure I could do at home. We were able to visit, but we were in a holding pattern, waiting.

On Monday, we met with a social worker. She asked a lot of questions about Alex, the family, his brother and sister, his friends in school, and what we thought about his emotional condition. I told her that Alex had seemed to deteriorate on the Zoloft, which he'd now been taking for several weeks. The angry outbursts had become more frequent and more severe. He threatened suicide often. The social worker had asked Alex many of the same questions, trying to put together a history that could help lead to a diagnosis. Alex told her he could not remember his angry outbursts when they were over, that he often felt sleepy afterward. He said that during one recent outburst he had heard two voices, one telling him to stop and the other to continue. He said he had experienced mood swings that lasted up to a day, teetering from depression to wild elation. These had become more common during the preceding two weeks, he said. He was given a battery of routine blood and urine tests; all were normal, the social worker said.

Alex had also been examined by one of the hospital psychiatrists. Taking a different approach from Alex's first psychiatrist, this one wanted to rule out the possibility that Alex's behavior was the result of some kind of seizure. Psychiatrist No. 2 consulted a neurologist, who suggested that Alex be given a "sleep-deprived EEG," a brain-wave reading done after he'd been kept awake all night, so that unusual brain activity might be more likely to show up. He also ordered a CT scan (what used to be called a CAT scan) of Alex's head. The hospital staff had monitored Alex closely throughout the day, looking for any indication he might try to hurt himself. They saw none. Alex kept to himself in the morning, but by the afternoon was participating in group therapy sessions and recreational activities, the social worker reported. A nurse asked Alex whether he had had any traumatic experiences. "Probably being in here is the worst thing that ever happened to me," he said.

Psychiatrist No. 2 had started Alex on Tegretol, a medication first used to treat seizures and now prescribed for a variety of psychiatric ailments. Uncertain whether Alex was suffering from a seizure disorder or a psychiatric illness, he was covering both possibilities with a drug that might be helpful in either case. I began to get a sense of how imprecise and subjective psychiatric treatment can be. Psychiatrists mix and match medicines for all kinds of reasons. Occasionally they have scientific evidence to back up these treatment decisions, but more often they are acting on experience, because the appropriate scientific studies have not been done. Some medicines are used for so many psychiatric ailments that I wonder whether they have any effect at all.

The social worker closed her file, stood, grabbed her keys from the desktop, and led us down the hallway to see Alex. She unlocked the door to the ward, waited as we followed her in, and turned to lock the door behind her. Alex was in the common room with a dozen other kids. He dropped what he was doing and came over to give Liz and me a hug. He looked sad. When we asked him why, he said, "There's nothing to talk about." We spoke briefly. None of us had much to say. It was tough to make conversation when all we could think about was what was wrong and when he was coming home. Alex wandered into another room, where the rest of the patients were watching a movie. He took a folding chair near some of the other kids and moved it away before sitting down. He sat alone, refusing to talk to the staff or the other kids. We said good night and left him there.

Alex was a little agitated that night and was having trouble falling asleep. He was given Benadryl, the allergy medication. Its drawback as an allergy medicine is that it induces sleepiness. In psychiatric hospitals, it's prescribed for precisely that reason, as a mild sleep inducer. The next day Alex participated in all of the group's activities. But each time, he started in a chair at the edge of the group, and then slowly joined the discussion and moved closer. He talked about how much he hated school. He complained about the arguments between Liz and me. "I'm afraid they will get divorced," he said. When asked whether he had any good qualities, he said, "I'm kind to my dog."

On his third day in the hospital, Alex became agitated. He spent the morning in the "quiet room," a small room used to confine patients who become angry or agitated and cannot be soothed, to ensure that they don't hurt themselves. A quiet room is empty except for a mattress on the floor. Left alone there, some children are able to calm themselves. Some require sedation. Alex was released after lunch, protesting that he had not done anything to deserve confinement. During one of the three, hour-long periods each day during which patients were allowed to call home, Alex called his mother to complain about his treatment. He got angry with her and hung up. He was again sent to the quiet room. He banged on the door, demanding to be let out. The staff tried to work with him, to find out what was wrong. But he refused to talk to them.

The next day was a good day, and we all knew that was important, because good behavior counted toward getting him out of there. The cause of his "recovery" was as mysterious as the cause of his outbursts the day before. He was cooperative and remorseful. The hospital staff said he'd taken an interest in some of the younger patients, and was helping them adjust to the hospital. He was doing so well on this, his fourth day in the hospital, that the staff began to plan for his discharge. They had made no progress in diagnosing Alex's condition. The hospital was having some sort of scheduling problem, and he still had not had the EEG or the CT scan that had been ordered the first day but could not be done on the weekend. I was afraid that he would be discharged without those tests, and that we might miss a critical clue about the cause of his distress. I was afraid that his behavior might be the result of some sort of atypical seizure disorder or, worse, a brain tumor, and that he would be discharged before it was found. Maybe it was something that could be cured if dealt with quickly. I was assured that the tests would be done. Alex's social worker scheduled a family therapy session for the next day.

I left work early for the two-hour train trip to the Boonton Township station, near the hospital but too far to walk. Liz was supposed to pick me up at the station on her way to the hospital. Somehow, we had crossed signals, and she went directly to the hospital. While I was standing on the platform, fretting over the time and wondering what had happened, the social worker canceled the family therapy session, because I wasn't there. Liz found me at the train station an hour later. We argued about who had been responsible for the missed connection. The family therapy session was not rescheduled. Alex had had his sleep-deprived EEG and CT scan, and both were normal. He was scheduled to be discharged on Friday, April 26, one week after being admitted.

Alex beamed when he was told he would be leaving. It was easy to forget the state he'd been in only a week earlier. He looked much stronger. The dark circles were gone from his eyes, and he was eager to see his brother and sister. He wanted to see Reggie, our Scottish Terrier. He told the staff that he had learned a lot about himself during his stay, and they were pleased with his improvement. He said the hospital stay had helped him and he expected to do much better at home and at school after his discharge. We drove him home, bought him pizza, and celebrated his return. It was like welcoming him home from summer camp. I was relieved, and happy to have him home, and I set my worries aside for the evening.

But they returned the next day. Alex still had no diagnosis. He had had only minimal therapy, a session or two a day for less than a week. When he was discharged, he had been on Tegretol for three days, far too little time to determine whether it was helping. It was tempting to believe that the problem had been solved. But I was skeptical. I couldn't see how such a short stay in the hospital could do much of anything. The hospital had kept Alex safe, when he needed to be kept safe, and Liz and I had had a chance to talk about Alex with Psychiatrist No. 2 and a social worker. But they didn't have any answers. We had a long, thoughtful conversation with the neurologist, who said he didn't think Alex had a seizure disorder or a brain tumor, but that he would need more tests if we wanted to be certain.

The hospital discharged Alex on the condition that he continue to receive psychiatric treatment, but didn't direct us to anyone who could provide that treatment. Psychiatrist No. 2 had undone the work of the first psychiatrist Alex had seen, dropping the Zoloft in favor of Tegretol. I started to keep score: this was Alex's third drug, after a total of three visits to two psychiatrists. Each visit seemed to generate a new hypothesis and a new treatment. I didn't know anything about how psychiatric diagnoses or treatment decisions were made, but this seemed wrong. I wanted to get Alex set up with a good child psychiatrist who could spend some time with him, get to know him, and make a treatment decision based on more than twenty or thirty minutes of conversation. The hospital staff agreed. But when I asked whether they could recommend a good psychiatrist for us, they said,

Sorry, we don't know any in your area. So what now? I asked the hospital staff. Where will we go for help? We really wish we could help you, the kindly social worker said; Alex is such a bright boy. Best of luck.

With no child psychiatrists on the insurance company's preferred-provider list, we had to abandon the list. We asked Alex's school psychologist to help. He recommended that we take Alex to see a local psychiatrist who knew our community and its children. We made an appointment. Psychiatrist No. 3.

Alex seemed fine during the first weekend after his discharge, except for an episode of uncontrollable laughter. On Monday morning, however, he refused to go to school. "I'm not going. Get away from me!" he shouted at his mother. He pulled his hair, thrashed around on the bed, and eventually calmed down and fell into a deep sleep. He spent most of the day in bed. His outbursts were often followed by a deep, trancelike sleep, after which he couldn't recall what had happened.

Psychiatrist No. 3 had a large number of patients with attention-deficit/hyperactivity disorder, or ADHD, one of the most common brain disorders in children. He was treating many of them with Ritalin. After his visit with Alex, Psychiatrist No. 3 concluded that Alex, too, was suffering from ADHD. He stopped the Tegretol and started Alex on Ritalin. He added Ativan, an antianxiety drug that he thought might help with the more ferocious emotional swings. But Alex's condition began to deteriorate as soon as he started taking the medication. His outbursts became more frequent and more severe. It seemed to me that these psychiatrists were diagnosing a complex emotional problem and dispensing medication with no more care or deliberation than if they were swabbing Alex's throat for strep and sending him away with penicillin. I updated my tally: three psychiatrists, four visits, four drugs. All within less than two months.

I'm not sure why it seemed so crucial to get Alex a proper diagnosis. Partly, I suppose, it was because I wanted to get him the right treatment, and I wanted to know what his prognosis was. Would he get better? Would he struggle with this for the rest of his life? Without a diagnosis, it was hard to know what to think.

Much later, I learned that proper diagnosis is not easy. "Diagnosis in psychiatry is a problem" and "distinguishing between normal behaviors and pathological ones in a young child is even more challenging," writes Dr. Demitri Papolos, a psychiatrist in Connecticut and the coauthor, with his wife, Janice, of *The Bipolar Child*. Children are constantly changing, developing, and growing, so it's hard to compare their lives before the onset of illness with their lives afterward. And it can be hard to sit them down for a thoughtful conversation. "Children are often misdiagnosed," they write, or plastered "with a literal alphabet soup of diagnostic labels: attention-deficit disorder with hyperactivity (ADHD), obsessive-compulsive disorder (OCD), oppositional defiant disorder (ODD), conduct disorder (CD), generalized anxiety disorder (GAD), and so on."

In cardiology, a diagnosis can be as neat and quick as the snap of the needle on an electrocardiograph. But there is no measure for depression, no blood test to identify schizophrenia or mania. In psychiatry, diagnoses overlap and flow into one another, blurring like the colors on an artist's palette. Instead of making a diagnosis and then choosing a drug, it often seems that psychiatrists will choose a drug to help make a diagnosis. If a patient responds to lithium, she has bipolar disorder, otherwise known as manic depression. If she does better on an antipsychotic, she has schizophrenia. If a child seems calmer on Ritalin, he has attention-deficit/ hyperactivity disorder.

Psychiatrists disagree so often and so profoundly about their diagnoses that they have devised a cookbook of symptoms to help them out. This book, the *Diagnostic and Statistical Manual of Mental Disorders,* which is published by the American Psychiatric Association, is unlike anything you'll find in the office of a cardiologist or an oncologist. *DSM-IV,* as it's called (the current version is the fourth edition), lists psychiatric symptoms and reduces diagnosis to a complex multiple-choice quiz. You might think, for example, that diagnosing a manic episode in a person with bipolar disorder would be relatively simple. It seems easy enough to any parent who has had to help a child get through a manic episode. Not so for psychiatrists, however. In their zeal to make their diagnoses accurate, they have devised elaborate checklists that exclude many patients who need help. *DSM-IV* lists five criteria for a manic episode, for example. This is the second of the five, with its seven subsidiary benchmarks:

> During the period of mood disturbance, three (or more) of the following symptoms have persisted (four if the mood is only irritable) and have been present to a significant degree:
>
> 1. inflated self-esteem or grandiosity
> 2. decreased need for sleep (e.g., feels rested after only 3 hours of sleep)
> 3. more talkative than usual or pressure to keep talking

4. flight of ideas or subjective experience that thoughts are racing
5. distractibility (i.e., attention too easily drawn to unimportant or irrelevant external stimuli)
6. increase in goal-directed activity (either socially, at work or school, or sexually) or psychomotor agitation
7. excessive involvement in pleasurable activities that have a high potential for painful consequences (e.g., engaging in unrestrained buying sprees, sexual indiscretions, or foolish business investments)

A child with three of these satisfies one of the five principal criteria for mania. Only two, and he doesn't. *DSM-IV* also includes a sly acknowledgment, in the small print of a footnote, that doctors trying to diagnose mania can just as easily cause it: "Note: Manic-like episodes that are clearly caused by somatic antidepressant treatment (e.g., medication, electroconvulsive therapy, light therapy) should not count toward a diagnosis," it says. In other words, if the mania was caused by something a psychiatrist administered during the trial-and-error phase of treatment, it was not really mania. It was a mistake. What *DSM-IV* doesn't do is remind doctors to apologize to these patients.

I didn't know any of this when we were first dealing with Alex's difficulties. And because we'd never been given a good explanation of what was happening to Alex, I continued to believe that he was not suffering from a real psychiatric illness. Maybe what he needed was a change of friends. Around the time that Alex's outbursts worsened, he had stopped seeing a boy who had been his best friend for several years. I didn't know why, and Alex wouldn't explain. But he did explain to Psychiatrist No. 3, the one who had prescribed

Ritalin. Apparently, the friend had been starting to spend less time with Alex and more time with another boy. Alex confronted his friend on the playground, and punched him. Other kids then descended upon Alex, surrounding him and hitting him. The pummeling didn't hurt as much as the loneliness afterward, Alex told Psychiatrist No. 3. Alex said he'd lost several friends, one after the other. In every case, he said, he became angry and picked a fight. It frightened Alex. He didn't know why it kept happening, or what to do about it. Until he'd talked to the psychiatrist, he hadn't shared his fears with anyone. The psychiatrist asked Alex to make three wishes. "I'd like to be reborn, so I could start all over again," Alex said. The psychiatrist waited; Alex was quiet. He didn't use his two other wishes.

The day after this visit, Alex was agitated and depressed, and getting worse by the hour. Maybe it was time to think about putting Alex in the hospital, said Psychiatrist No. 3. He suggested we call 911 if things got any worse. I wanted to know why he wasn't arranging for Alex's possible admission to a hospital. What was the point of having psychiatric care if in an emergency the psychiatrist wasn't involved? I didn't want Alex sent to the county hospital, and that's what would have happened if we'd called 911. Instead, we insisted that the psychiatrist see Alex again. He set up an emergency appointment two days later. The psychiatrist found him resistant to treatment, mistrustful, and hostile, but Alex did start talking. He said he'd felt depressed "all my life," and now he felt even worse. The psychiatrist told us to stop the Ritalin, use the Ativan if necessary, and advised us again to call 911 if Alex seemed to present a danger to himself or anyone else.

Psychiatrist No. 3 was abandoning us. So I began calling

everyone I could think of for help. A friend, a lawyer with a hospital in New York, put me in touch with a psychiatrist colleague who gave me the names of people he thought were among the best child psychiatrists in New York. I told him I was concerned that if Alex were hospitalized again, he would once again be discharged too soon, before he had made any progress. "You have to fight," the psychiatrist told me. "Make it a risk-management issue. Deluge the hospital with the information showing he's a risk. Put the hospital on notice." The insurance company might have an arrangement in which any blame for inadequate care is shifted to the hospital, away from the insurance company, so the idea was to put pressure on the hospital. If they were worried about a malpractice suit, he said, they would fight with the insurance company to keep Alex there. "These people are not unprincipled," he said. "They want to do the right thing"; but to make that happen, I would have to put pressure on them.

I called one of the psychiatrists he referred me to. The man was on his way out of town and could speak to me only briefly. He gave me the name of another psychiatrist, a friend of his who might help; I spoke to him. I called a friend at Johns Hopkins University, who said she could put me in touch with a child psychiatrist there, if I wanted to bring Alex to Baltimore. I called the headquarters of the National Alliance for the Mentally Ill, a leading patient advocacy group, and was referred to a local representative. I called the insurance company to find out what kind of coverage I had for Alex, and I was told that only fifteen days would be covered at the full rate. After that, the insurance company would pay 70 percent of the hospital costs; I would be responsible for hundreds of dollars in charges per day after the first fifteen days. Alex had already been hospitalized seven days; I had only eight more days before my out-of-pocket costs would begin to skyrocket.

Within a few days, the angry outbursts had become almost constant. Liz called Psychiatrist No. 3, and he increased the dosage of Ritalin. That night, Alex had what seemed to be a reaction to the increased dose of medication. He was very disturbed and wouldn't respond to anything we said. He threatened suicide. We tried to get him to take a dose of Ativan, which was supposed to calm him in a crisis, but he wouldn't take it.

I called the psychiatrist. A woman at his answering service said he was not available. I pleaded with her to call him, saying we had an emergency on our hands. The psychiatrist called back a few minutes later to say there was nothing he could do. I'd been told I would have to fight, and this seemed like the time to start. If anything happened to Alex, I said, I would make it very clear that the psychiatrist had been contacted and had refused to help. I called the police. They said all they could do was to take Alex to the county hospital. Alex slipped further out of control. He still refused to take the Ativan. An hour later, Psychiatrist No. 3 called back to say he was trying to find a hospital bed for Alex.

By the next morning, Psychiatrist No. 3 had arranged for Alex's admission to the Westchester Division of the New York Hospital–Cornell Medical Center (now known as New York–Presbyterian) in White Plains, thirty miles north of New York City. He also made multiple calls to the insurance company, which demanded information on Alex's condition from the hospital before agreeing to cover Alex's treatment, then refused to precertify Alex's treatment because the hospital had not provided enough information on him. This was no surprise, because no one at the hospital had seen Alex yet. But, if Alex was not precertified, we might find later that we would have to pay for the hospital ourselves. Our entire savings would not have covered more than a few days. The psychiatrist called the insurance company again and informed them that Alex presented a danger to others and possibly to himself. That did the trick. He called the hospital to let them know Alex was on his way.

When Alex woke up that morning, he paced from room to room, refusing to take any medication and threatening me and Liz. Without letting Alex see her, Liz quietly packed a small suitcase for him to take to the hospital. She put it in the storage area behind the backseat of the minivan we owned then. When we got the call in late morning that Alex had been approved for admission, we told him that we were taking him to see a new psychiatrist. After much arguing and cajoling, we persuaded him to get in the car. He sat in the back; Liz drove, and I sat in the front passenger seat. It was about a forty-five-minute ride to the hospital. Five minutes after we left the house, Alex turned to look behind the backseat, saw the suitcase, and figured out where we were headed. We were on I-95 when he reached for the door and said he was going to jump out of the car. There was no place to pull over. Alex looked as though he meant it. I undid my seat belt, climbed between the front seats, and fell on top of Alex, pinning him to the seat. He screamed, punched, and kicked, trying to push me off of him. I pressed harder. I was stronger than he was, but not by much. We stayed that way until we pulled up in front of the hospital. Liz opened the door. I lifted myself off Alex, whose energy was mostly spent, and stepped unsteadily out of the car. I was exhausted, physically and emotionally. I wondered whether Alex would ever trust me again.

It was Wednesday, May 8, 1996, less than two weeks after his discharge from the first hospital. In the interim, he'd had two visits with Psychiatrist No. 3, who had prescribed Ritalin. Psychiatrist No. 3 had no professional connection with the new hospital, so Alex would be starting treatment with yet another new psychiatrist. The hospital was housed in dark brick buildings spread across grassy, wooded hills, which gave it the look of a small college. We stepped into a paneled hallway and signed in at the admissions desk. We waited with Alex for a tense half hour before a hospital staff member escorted us to the teenage unit, where Alex would stay until a bed opened up on the children's unit. On the way, he became increasingly agitated. "Take me home!" he yelled. Two aides ran up to him. He told them there was nothing wrong with him, that Liz and I were making up stories about what he'd done. They half-carried him to the quiet room and locked him inside. I could hear Alex banging against the door and the walls. The hospital staff assured us that they would take over and that Alex would be fine, and they pointed Liz and me toward the door. There was nothing we could do, no reason to stay. Get in the car and go home, they said. As we walked down a long empty corridor, Alex's agonized screams echoed off the walls. I could hear them until we reached the end of the corridor and walked through a large double door. I can hear them still.

The hospital gave him fifty milligrams of Benadryl to put him to sleep. When he woke up, the hospital staff began to address its immediate goals for Alex. The first was to soothe his anger and the physical abuse, threats, and resistance to treatment that went along with it. That night, and on the nights to follow, he was scheduled for observation checks every fifteen minutes until morning. The next day, he was tearful but able to calm himself and take a shower in the morning. By the afternoon, he began to talk to some of the other children in the unit. We visited him later that day, and he became somewhat agitated again, requiring another fifty milligrams of Benadryl. The hospital psychiatrist and the staff discussed whether Alex might be suffering from a disruptive behavior disorder, but eventually settled on bipolar disorder as the admitting diagnosis. It was the first time anyone had suggested this as the cause of his suffering.

We visited Alex every day. Liz drove from New Jersey, and I took the train from New York. One afternoon, before visiting hours had begun, I spotted Alex outside in a small, sunny courtyard, a little monastic hideaway in the middle of the children's unit. He was alone, at a small table, reading. I saw him through an open window, and called to him. He looked up and broke into a huge smile when he saw me. Oddly, it was in the otherwise difficult and sometimes tense circumstances of the hospital that we had some of our warmest exchanges. Alex's worst emotional breaks, the episodes that took him to the hospital, were followed by what was beginning to be a pattern. He would protest violently upon arrival at the hospital, saying he didn't belong here, that he was being unfairly punished for something that wasn't his fault. Whatever had happened was the fault of his teachers, or his parents, or the police, or anyone but him. Then he would begin to realize that he was going to be in the hospital no matter how strongly he argued against it, and he would embrace the treatment program. Within a day or two, he would become not only a model patient, but a favorite of the hospital staff. His worst days, in other words, were followed by his best.

On these visits, I brought books to read to him. Sometimes he read to us. We brought him Chinese food or a pizza to share. One of the nicest things about visiting hours, for Alex, was the chance to eat something other than hospital food. And we would talk about what had been bothering him, about how therapy was going, about his favorites on the staff, about what video was scheduled for that evening. The hospital had provided a safe place for Alex to let go of the emotions that were turning him inside out. But two or three days was still too short a time for any treatment the hospital provided to take effect. Alex's sudden improvement seemed to have more to do with him. He knew he was safe, he was in a highly structured, predictable environment, and he knew that if he behaved well he could go home soon. So he behaved well. I did not understand how simple, straightforward changes in Alex's environment could produce such a remarkable improvement so quickly. I no longer needed convincing that Alex was indeed suffering from some sort of emotional illness, although no one seemed to know exactly what it was. His outbursts were not the actions of a bad kid, or a kid who needed punishment. They were out of his control, the consequence of some medical condition that he could not change and that was causing him enormous suffering. But if this was a true psychiatric illness, how could it be controlled so readily by a change in circumstances?

It had taken Alex about three days to feel this comfortable. He was doing well, but he was burning through the days allotted by the insurance company, and we still didn't have a definitive diagnosis or a treatment plan. I was concerned that we would repeat what had happened with the first hospitalization, that Alex would seem fine, be released, and then descend into the same confusion and emotional distress that had plagued him for months. I called the hospital and explained my concern. What were they doing? I tried to tell them that each day was crucial, that Alex should be evaluated and should be seeing a psychiatrist regularly. The clock was ticking, I said, and I thought they should understand that.

Why was it so hard to explain this to them? Wasn't this a situation they faced all the time? Hours, sometimes a whole day, would go by when it seemed that Alex would be doing nothing but participating in loosely organized group therapy sessions, playing games, making a feeble effort to look at his schoolwork, or eating and sleeping. Where was the intervention that would really help him? I made these concerns known as forcefully as I could. When I didn't get much response, I tried calling the hospital's executives to demand that more be done. Desperate, I told them I would make sure that they did what they were supposed to do, and that if they didn't, I would resort to legal means to make certain that they did. It was an empty threat. I didn't have the energy or the financial resources to pursue a legal claim, and I knew I probably wouldn't have much of a case anyway. The simple truth was that I was angry. I wanted Alex to get better, and I was going to do whatever I could to make sure the hospital and its staff gave him all the help and attention he needed.

After the first few bright days at the hospital, Alex began to have problems. He was having trouble sleeping. It was the same problem he'd been having at home, sleeping erratically, sometimes staying awake all night and sleeping all day, or sleeping on and off at all hours. He did not seem well. His face was sallow. A nurse at the hospital noted that he had dark circles under his eyes. He was quiet, depressed, and apathetic, although he was able to avoid any violent outbursts. The hospital psychiatrist—for Alex, this was Psychiatrist No. 4—arranged for us to take Alex out on passes, for a couple of hours at a time, to the local mall to play video games and get something to eat. Although the psychiatrist didn't tell us so at the time, the idea was to see whether the violent episodes recurred during the time away from the hospital. They didn't. Whatever Alex's condition in the hospital ward, he was fine when he was with us. As with the first hospitalization, it was tempting to conclude that Alex was magically improving, even though not much was being done at the hospital. They did put him on lithium, a mood stabilizer and one of the most common treatments for bipolar disorder. We were told that this would help ease the emotional swings that seemed to be driving Alex's rage and depression.

On his sixth day in the hospital, Alex told the nurses that he felt like a failure, and that he had little hope of changing that. He no longer seemed violent, but he continued to need encouragement to interact with the other kids. He didn't take care of himself. He refused to comb his hair or to take showers; he skipped meals and complained of insomnia. Although he seemed much improved during the time Liz and I spent with him, he was doing poorly during the day when we were not there. And he was due to be discharged the next day; after that came the sharp drop in reimbursement. A representative of the insurance company recommended that Alex be transferred to a part-time hospital program. She was not a psychiatrist, and, more important, she had never met Alex. Yet she was suggesting a change that would profoundly affect his medical care, and possibly, if his feelings of worthlessness and despair continued, his life. And what would be my recourse if Alex were discharged and something tragic occurred? There would be none. The insurance company was within its rights, according to its contract with my employer, to refuse additional care.

A social worker at the hospital gamely tried to find a part-time hospital program for Alex. There was no alternative. She talked to administrators at two such programs in New Jersey. Both said Alex was too young for their programs, and neither knew of any other in the state of New Jersey that could accommodate an eleven-year-old boy. The hospital prepared a tentative discharge plan. Alex would return home, and would return to the care of Psychiatrist No. 3, who had prescribed the Ritalin that appeared to have sent Alex into a tailspin. It didn't seem like much of a plan to me, and I said so. I insisted that we could not return to the same psychiatrist. I had been favorably impressed by the psychiatrist at the hospital. It was an academic institution, affiliated with Cornell University's medical school in New York City, and the staff seemed better educated and more aware of current psychiatric research and practice than the psychiatrists Alex had seen elsewhere. I asked whether Alex could continue to see the psychiatrist who was treating him at the hospital. No, the hospital staff did not provide outpatient care. There would be no exceptions. When the social worker told the insurance company that no part-time hospitalization program was available for Alex, the insurance company operative told the hospital that she would review the case and call with her decision the next day—the day Alex was scheduled to be discharged.

The night before the scheduled discharge, we went to the hospital for a parent-child group meeting, meant to be comforting and instructive. I found it tiresome. I had too much on my mind to be willing to show interest in the problems of others, and I was short on insights. Alex said he was having bad dreams at the hospital, dreams that scared him, but he didn't say what they were. A nurse explained to Liz a point system that she could use with Alex at home, a way to reward good behavior with privileges, not unlike what was done in the hospital. The next morning, the insurance company called to say that it was granting Alex two more days at the hospital, and that it would review his case again then. The hospital staff found that Alex was still depressed, distant, and apathetic. He was still having trouble sleeping, and he didn't have much of an appetite. For the first time, Alex was sent to participate in the children's unit school program in the morning. In group therapy that afternoon, he said that in school he tried to be the class clown to impress his friends. He started acting silly in the group and tried to encourage the other patients to join him, but he was "easily redirected," the hospital staff reported. "Underlying low self-esteem appears to be at the core of his difficulties," according to a report by his psychiatrist, who observed him in the group setting. "He feels he is unable to make friends by just being himself," and he "has a nihilistic view of the world." The word "nihilistic" stayed with me. I could imagine an adult having a nihilistic view of the world, but I was taken aback to hear the word applied to my eleven-year-old boy, the child with the warm heart and easy smile.

We had a family meeting at the hospital the next

morning. I was skeptical of the value of these sessions, and while I tried to be open and honest, I didn't feel that they were contributing much to Alex's treatment. I worried that they would open wounds and unleash a barrage of grievances. The children had long-standing gripes with one another and with Liz and me, and communication between Liz and me hadn't improved. I was afraid that we would merely allow angry feelings to escape without time to resolve them. In the end, not much happened in the session. It had become distressingly clear to me that stress, anger, and anxiety surged through our family in a tangle of jagged nerves. Perhaps this had caused Alex's difficulties; it had certainly contributed to them. It was also clear that this wouldn't be easy to resolve. The family session led us nowhere.

The next morning, Alex was sent home.

Psychiatrist No. 3 was unwilling to take Alex back as a patient. Perhaps he felt he could do no more, or maybe he didn't want to see me again, after I'd threatened legal action. The insurance company, in one brief empathetic gasp before Alex's discharge, had given us the name of a psychiatrist to monitor Alex's medication, and a psychologist to provide therapy.

Although the hospital psychiatrist had tentatively given Alex a diagnosis of bipolar disorder, neither he nor anyone else on the staff seemed sure that was correct. The new tally: four psychiatrists, none of whom Alex had seen for more than two or three visits, and his fifth drug, lithium. He had not been on any one medication for more than two weeks. Although he seemed better to Liz and me, he continued to experience periods of depression. There was no way to know whether the threats and the violent behavior at home and at school would return. We had exhausted our allotment of hospital days covered by the insurance company. If Alex were hospitalized again, we would be responsible for a substantial portion of the cost ourselves. We didn't know what the future held. We knew only one thing: Alex was suffering. We all were.

CHAPTER THREE

When I was a child, in the fifties, my parents used to tell me that I could grow up to be president of the United States. We thought anything was possible. Some parents might not choose a career in politics for their children now, but we still cherish the belief, as we cradle them, that they can grow up to be or do almost anything. My mother and father had worked hard to give me opportunities that they hadn't had. I had planned to do the same for my children. I had never imagined that raising them could become a life-and-death struggle, but now I found myself fighting to keep Alex alive. Any other thoughts about what he might one day accomplish fell away as Liz and I focused on getting him through each day, through each week, through the last couple of months of fifth grade.

During those last months, from April through June, Alex rarely attended school. He was still sleeping erratically, often up for hours at night, and therefore having difficulty getting out of bed in the morning. He rarely had the energy for school, and he often teetered between one difficult emotion and another. His teacher continued to treat him not as a sick child, but as a bad kid. When Alex was in the hospital in

Westchester, she called the social worker there to warn her
about him, to tell her that he might try to disrupt his hospital ward as he had his classroom. Alex would "target a peer
and recruit his friends to terrorize the child," the teacher
said. It was bizarre behavior for a teacher. I could understand
why Alex refused to go to school.

It was during Alex's second hospitalization that the social
worker, school psychologist, and others who had been eval-
uating Alex at the principal's suggestion completed their
report. By now, I understood the importance of the evaluation by the child-study team. The idea was to determine
whether Alex should be classified as a special education student under state law. Such a classification would do two
things. It would make him eligible for extra help and special
classes, something he clearly would need, at least for a while.
And it would, in some sense, separate him from the other
kids. For children classified as special education students, a
line had been drawn between those who were considered
normal and those who were not.

On May 14, the child-study team determined that Alex
was eligible for special education, and the extra help that
went with that. To classify him as a special education student, the team had to put him in one of several categories, as
specified by the state. Some students received special services
because of handicaps or neurological impairments. Children
with psychiatric ailments were lumped together as "emotionally disturbed," a term that felt cold and harsh. Alex was
not "emotionally disturbed." He was not abnormal, or different. He was a normal child who had an illness that affected
his moods. The term seemed to confuse the child with the
disease.

In its report, the child-study team once again affirmed

that Alex's performance in school was falling far short of his ability. His verbal IQ was 122, and his full-scale IQ was 114. He was capable of doing well in school, and some days he did. But he took little satisfaction from the good days. He was convinced that he wasn't succeeding, even when he was doing well.

Most days, after he returned from his second hospitalization, he didn't go to school at all, or he left at lunchtime. When he was in school, he would frequently leave the classroom without permission and head for the principal's office, which now felt like a haven to him. "I was so different," Alex told me much later, when I asked him about the early years of his illness. "Who else had the cops come and pick them up in fifth grade?" Part of the reason he played sports, he said, was to show that he was good at something, "to show that I was something other than that crazy kid at school."

In June, the child-study team presented Liz and me with a draft of Alex's individualized education program, or IEP. The IEP spells out the educational program that the school has determined is best for the student. Parents are free to challenge the IEP's adequacy and appropriateness, and to suggest changes. Liz and I did neither. At that point, we had no idea what was right for him. We read the IEP and signed it. Under its terms, Alex would be sent to a private, out-of-district school, where he would receive much closer supervision and, we hoped, a better education. If he did well there in the sixth grade, he would be brought back to Ridgewood the following year, back to the middle school for seventh grade.

The problem was, what school would he go to? Schools for special education students fall into a couple of categories.

Some are for students with clear, diagnosed learning disabilities and such conditions as attention-deficit/hyperactivity disorder, which require special instructional methods. Alex did not fall into that category. He was an intelligent and capable student. Other schools are aimed at children with neurological impairments, sensory deficits, or other physical handicaps. Alex did not fit into that category, either. The child-study team suggested that we look at a few schools in the area. Alex wasn't happy to hear that he would not be attending the Ridgewood middle school the following year with his friends and classmates. But we wanted him to have a say in which school he attended, so we took him along on the visits. We were all upset with the choices. Alex had endured a terrible year in fifth grade, and there was every reason to expect that things would get worse in the sixth grade if he moved to the Ridgewood middle school, which was bigger and less closely supervised than his elementary school. But I couldn't quite picture him with the kids we saw in the schools we visited. And none of the schools seemed right. Some were dreary and dark, others ramshackle and poorly maintained. Alex didn't like any of them, and neither did I.

After we had been at this for a few weeks, we heard about a school with an energetic director who had left an executive position in the state education department to operate several private schools for special ed students. He and the schools were highly regarded, as far as we could tell. We put Alex in the car and paid a visit.

The school, half an hour's drive from home, occupied what had once been a large department store, on the main street of a small town. From the outside, it looked like a refurbished department store. But inside, it was sunny, open, and quite pleasant. It had new classrooms, fresh paint, and a personable and energetic staff. It was the first place we'd seen that didn't make my shoulders sag. We met the director in the gym, where he shot a few baskets with Alex before taking us into his office to tell us a little bit about the school. Its students were bright kids who needed smaller classes and more individualized instruction, but they weren't handicapped, he said. That seemed like a good fit for Alex. The school would not take him, however, if he did not want to go there. The director excused Liz and me from his office, and asked Alex to come in, alone. I didn't expect Alex to go with him, but he did. Twenty minutes later, the director emerged with Alex and said he thought our son would do well there. "This is a kid I can work with," he said. We had a deal.

The tuition was in the neighborhood of $20,000 per year, far beyond what we could afford. But we didn't have to pay it. The school system, obligated to provide an education for all students in the district, was required to pick up the tab for educational programs that it could not provide. To their credit, school officials never hesitated over the question of paying the tuition. That was one of the virtues of living in a wealthy town, with a financially healthy school district. Parents in poorer communities often have to fight for the rights that are supposed to be guaranteed to them by federal law. We didn't have to do that. As I later realized, Ridgewood was eager to move students with problems out of the district and into private schools, despite the costs. The town's educational programs were directed toward the upwardly mobile children of its upper-middle-class clientele. The Ridgewood schools had neither the time nor the inclination to devote special help to students with educational or emotional difficulties. It is much easier, and, in the end, cheaper, to send them away.

Alex missed a lot of classes during the rest of the fifth grade, but he managed to get through the year, and his condition seemed to be improving. The hospital had given us the names of several psychiatrists in our area. We had chosen one who was covered by our insurance. This was Psychiatrist No. 5. Amazingly, he did not begin by starting Alex on a new drug, as all the others had. He continued Alex on lithium (Drug No. 5), which the hospital had prescribed. Bipolar disorder was still the working diagnosis, but no one seemed ready to declare, with any confidence, that the case was closed. Lithium, a treatment for bipolar disorder, seemed to be working moderately well, and that was as far as anyone would go.

Lithium is a tricky drug. If the dose is too low, it doesn't work. If the dose is too high, it can cause kidney damage. Psychiatrist No. 5 periodically ordered blood tests to make sure that the lithium circulating in Alex's system was within the safe and effective range. Otherwise, Psychiatrist No. 5 saw Alex rarely. His job was to dispense drugs and to make sure they were administered properly. Insurance companies don't like to pay psychiatrists for therapy, because they charge more than twice as much per hour as psychologists and social workers. Children (and adults) with mental illness typically have a psychiatrist to prescribe their medications, and a therapist to help them understand and cope with their illnesses. Often the psychiatrist and the therapist have never met, and they rarely talk. Neither one is entirely in charge of the patient's care. The therapist, who talks to the patient at length, is the one in a position to evaluate the patient, but it is the psychiatrist, who may have little familiarity with the patient's condition, who prescribes the drugs.

That was precisely the situation Alex was in. He was seeing a psychologist, whom we'd found with help from the hospital. It didn't seem to me that these weekly visits were helping Alex. I could hear him raging at the therapist as I sat outside in the waiting room. Occasionally, the therapist would ask me to come in. Alex was quieter while I was in the room, but the raging resumed when I left. I asked the therapist what was going on. "This is a place where he can say what he wants, and act the way he wants, and feel safe," he said. "This is his space." I think Alex was smarter than the therapist. I think Alex was trying to push him to the point at which he would dismiss Alex from his care. Alex didn't like therapy, he didn't think he needed it, and he didn't think it was helping. It's possible that a change in Alex's medication might have helped him remain calm during sessions. Perhaps if he'd taken something to relax him before the sessions, the therapy would have been far more productive. At the time, it didn't occur to me to ask the psychiatrist. I had no relationship with him, and he wasn't available for extended discussions about Alex's treatment. He didn't get paid for that. So we drifted. After a few months of angry arguments in the therapist's office, Alex refused to go. He had won his battle with the therapist. I didn't see the point of continuing these fruitless sessions, and I didn't have the energy to begin the search for a new therapist. We dropped the therapy. The daily doses of lithium were his only treatment.

Nevertheless, as summer began, Alex seemed to unclench his hands and his jaw for the first time in months.

There were fewer crises. He finished school and he had a pleasant summer. I was as confused as ever.

In September 1996, a small yellow bus began picking Alex up at the house each morning to take him to his new school. Within a couple of weeks, we saw clearly that it had been a good choice. Not only was Alex no longer a "problem kid," he was quickly emerging as a star. He did well in his classes, he participated in intramural sports, and he charmed everyone with whom he came into contact. This was the first time, I think, that Alex learned the full power of his charm. Freed, for at least a while, from the oppression of the emotional storms that had beset him in the spring, and away from the teacher who detested him, the real Alex began to emerge, the Alex that we had known from the time he was a baby. He got along well with the other students, but he kept them at a distance. He never invited any of them to his house to play, nor did he visit theirs. He continued to spend time after school with his friends in Ridgewood. It was important to him to not be defined as a kid who wasn't normal, a label that had been forced upon him.

He proved a diligent student, and his evaluations reflected that. "Alex reads with great fluency . . . is consistent in completing his assignments and enjoys reading for pleasure," his teacher wrote in November. He worked hard at spelling and writing, mastered math, participated eagerly in social studies discussions, and excelled in science. Sometimes he was slow in starting his assignments; he could become frustrated easily, and he was inconsistent in completing his homework. Occasionally he needed help remaining focused in the classroom. But these problems were mild, compared with the praise. With such encouragement and support, Alex seemed readily able to overcome his difficulties. The boy whom his fifth-grade teacher had described as a trouble-maker was now described as "a wonderful asset to the classroom," who "is respectful to his classmates and shows good teamwork." He "possesses good athletic ability" and "is a wonderfully talented young artist," his teachers wrote. "Alex is always pleasant and I enjoy having him in my class." This was the Alex I knew.

One observation in Alex's evaluation caught my eye. "He responds well to a structured setting and positive reinforcement," his homeroom teacher wrote. That was the key: a structured environment. The school used a behavior-modification system in which students collected points for good behavior. The students were also assigned to a "level" that reflected their behavior. Higher levels carried more privileges. Points could be redeemed at the school store for school supplies, items with the school logo, or even a basketball. Alex quickly built up his point total and rose to a level that granted him considerable leeway, although always within the context of the structured environment.

As the year went on, Alex began to flourish in other areas as well. He was "an excellent leader," and "one of the first students to hand in a long-term project and present it with confidence," a teacher said. He was repeatedly described as "a great team worker."

Alex's mood also improved, except for a shaky period in March, about a year after his hospitalizations. Spring, it seemed, was a difficult time for him. It's not unusual for people with mood disorders to experience a seasonal pattern in their moods. Many have trouble in the spring. No one is quite sure, however, why this occurs. Some studies suggest that temperature variations play a role. Others point to the change in day length between summer and winter.

That spring, Alex began seeing a new psychiatrist. A friend, a social worker who did therapy with children, knew of a child psychiatrist near Ridgewood who she thought was particularly good. It wasn't easy to get in to see him. His schedule was full, and he didn't often take new patients. But we persisted, and eventually were able to bring Alex in for an evaluation. Alex had been doing passably well with Psychiatrist No. 5, but he clearly needed more help. The new psychiatrist, No. 6, talked to Alex for more than an hour; then he asked Alex to sit in the waiting room while he took Liz and me into his office.

For the first time, we got an unambiguous diagnosis. Alex did indeed have bipolar disorder, Psychiatrist No. 6 said. He planned to continue prescribing lithium, which, he explained was a mood stabilizer, not an antidepressant; it would moderate the up-and-down mood swings of Alex's illness. Psychiatrist No. 6 also planned to begin regular therapy sessions with Alex, meaning that Alex's medical care and therapy would be coordinated. It seemed like a breakthrough. Finally, we'd found someone who seemed both competent and caring, and who was willing to devote his full attention to Alex. There was only one problem: He didn't accept insurance payments. We would need to pay for each session out of our own pockets, at a cost of $250 per hour. The insurance company might reimburse some of that, but we had no guarantee. It wasn't easy to make those payments. They amounted to $1,000 a month when Alex was seeing the psychiatrist regularly, more than we were paying for the mortgage on our house. But how could we say no?

It soon became clear that this had been the right decision. With the help of Psychiatrist No. 6, Alex managed to get through the spring without again requiring hospitalization.

In a standardized test given at the end of the year, Alex scored in the ninety-seventh percentile in reading and the ninetieth percentile nationally in math. It was a wonderful year for him. The growth in his confidence, his organizational ability, and his desire to succeed were impressive. And he was so much happier.

Indeed, he did so well that his teachers decided to send him back to the Ridgewood school system. In May, the Ridgewood schools evaluated Alex, in accordance with the requirements for special education students, and issued a report. "His emotional and behavioral difficulties have shown marked improvement," the report said. "Alex is currently receiving medication to control his mood swings, and it had proven successful." Academically, "Alex has continued to demonstrate strong ability. He is currently functioning at or above grade level in all areas. He completes independent assignments and projects in a timely fashion, and he works cooperatively in group situations." The report noted Alex's emotional growth, as well: "He is comfortable with his peers, shows respect for authority, and responds well to praise and encouragement." Finally, "continued cooperation between Alex, school staff, parents and psychiatrist would be essential to Alex's success at the middle school next year," and such cooperation was "an expected certainty." Alex "appears to warrant consideration for transfer to a less-restrictive setting for the 1997–1998 school year."

I'd like to say that Liz and I had the presence of mind to argue. But we didn't. I wanted Alex back in the regular schools. I wanted him to do well there; I wanted him to be happy. I wanted to make all of this go away, to put it behind us. *Let's just start clean. We are going to get through this.* Everyone thought Alex was in good shape. If anyone had suggested that it might be better for Alex to spend another year or two in the private school, I might have been able to see that that was a better plan. But without any dissent to grab on to, I was happy to take the unanimous advice of the professionals and send Alex back to Ridgewood.

Psychiatrist No. 6, who had been seeing Alex for only two months, enthusiastically supported the recommendation. The prevailing opinion was that his success in the private school, where he received close attention and support, signified that he no longer needed such attention. This didn't make a lot of sense, but I welcomed it, and was happy to overlook the skewed logic. Alex, like most children, wanted to be normal. He felt that he had earned the right to come back to the Ridgewood schools. That, he explained, had been the primary motivation behind his success. He'd done everything he was supposed to do, and he'd done it well, and he deserved to come back, he told us. He had a point. We had a contract, and he'd honored his end of it. Now we had to honor ours.

In the fall, Alex settled into seventh grade at the public school. He did well in all his classes, and there was no sign of the problems he'd had in fifth grade. He was once again the capable student he had been before. All his evaluations said he was above average and above grade level. He continued to see Psychiatrist No. 6 and the therapist he had started with in the spring of sixth grade. His diagnosis didn't change, but he showed little sign of bipolar disorder. He kept taking lithium. We now had a name for Alex's illness, and we appeared to have a solution.

He was fine until March, when he deteriorated almost overnight. The angry outbursts sprang back. Some days he was fine; on other days, it was almost impossible to speak to him. His grades plummeted, and he lost interest in school. He narrowly averted another trip to the hospital.

But he couldn't recover from the disruption in school. The middle school's child-study team decided to excuse him from most of his regular assignments. There was no thought of holding Alex back in the seventh grade. He had done well through much of the year, and he was too bright. He would be promoted to the eighth grade the following year, with the rest of his class. His psychiatrist didn't change Alex's prescription. We hoped that he would recover in school the following year.

By the time Alex began eighth grade, the worst symptoms of his illness had subsided. But he never recovered his equilibrium in school. He clowned around in class. He was flippant with his teachers and ignored detentions. His academic record deteriorated. He simply stopped doing homework. In the spring, he became agitated again, and we began to fear that he would need to be hospitalized again. He was becoming increasingly difficult to handle in school. It was a near repeat of fifth grade, though this time without the added burden of a malevolent teacher.

The school began calling, sometimes two or three times a week, asking us to pick Alex up and take him home. Liz, who worked in Ridgewood, was the one who had to do that. I was too far away, and too pressured by the job to even stop and think much about the situation. The principal, the child-study team, and Alex's teachers had no idea how to factor his illness into their disciplinary program. Recalling the success of the year at the private school, I told them to treat him as they would any kid: He's just like everyone else. If he deserves detention, give him detention. Bad behavior is still bad behavior, I argued. The school officials said they were unwilling to apply their regular disciplinary code to Alex. They wanted Liz and me to solve the problem. But we weren't with Alex in school. We didn't see what was happening, and, as I kept saying, it wasn't up to us to set classroom rules for him. We did what we could at home, and they had to handle the chore at school.

The dark circles that had signaled the onset of Alex's illness reappeared under his eyes. He held his head down, toward the ground, and rarely looked anyone in the eye. He threatened Liz, and less often me, saying he would hurt us if we got in his way. He regularly threatened to cut or kill himself.

By April, everyone agreed that Alex would need to be hospitalized. For the first time, I did not despair at the thought. Alex was talking about suicide. I was afraid we might lose him. Did he mean it? Who could tell? I couldn't, Alex's teachers couldn't, and by this time I didn't have much faith that any psychiatrist could, including Nos. 1 through 6. The memory of the sound of the door locking Alex inside the first hospital no longer made me despair. I just wanted him to be safe.

Toward the end of April, Alex found himself in the grip of his illness again, unable to govern his emotions. He left the school in late morning, apparently after some altercation with teachers, and the police set out to find him. He returned to school on his own. Later, I found an unsmoked package of cigarettes in his backpack; maybe he had gone out to buy them. When he returned to school, Alex was taken to the principal's office. He said he wanted to put a gun in his mouth.

The principal called and asked permission to have Alex picked up by the police; he said he could no longer guarantee Alex's safety. We agreed. Alex was taken to the police station. I left work and jumped on the train. We got to the police station a few hours later. Alex now seemed calm and fragile. An understanding officer, who often worked with kids, persuaded him to go to the emergency room. He put Alex in his car, and we followed. We arrived just after four P.M. The hospital began processing Alex for a temporary stay in the emergency room, until he could be transferred to a psychiatric hospital. But where? Psychiatrist No. 6 recommended Four Winds Hospital, in Katonah, New York, about ninety miles from Ridgewood. It was not clear whether Four Winds had a bed for Alex, but an emergency room nurse began to arrange for transportation anyway. It was difficult to find an ambulance. All ambulance services in the area were booked. And we weren't sure who would pay for it. A crisis counselor at the hospital had called my insurance company to arrange coverage for both the hospital admission and the ambulance transfer, but the insurance company had not called back. Nothing could happen until we got approval.

Alex, who had been relatively calm since we arrived at the emergency room, now began to get agitated again. He was leaving, he said. The illness was surging in him, building in intensity. A nurse called for help, and several aides held him down while they sedated him. He protested, but within minutes he slipped into unconsciousness. The hospital was not equipped to handle psychiatric emergencies. They'd given him the chemical equivalent of a locked door.

The effort to get approval from the insurance company

went on for several hours, and the insurance company still had not called back. Finally, I got on the phone to the insurance company and refused to hang up until the company returned the crisis counselor's call on another line. Alex had left school in the middle of the day. It was now eight P.M. I left to check on Alicia and Matt, who were home alone. What I really wanted to do was get out of the emergency room, and away from the grinding, glacial passage of time.

Around nine P.M., Four Winds said it had a bed for Alex, but we still had no ambulance, and transportation by ambulance was a requirement of the emergency room. We waited. Time crawled. I began to feel as if I'd been sedated myself.

From time to time during the evening, I had been distracted by news footage on the television screens suspended over patients' beds, showing frantic high school students running across a school lawn. I looked more closely at one of the TVs. It was April 20, 1999. That morning, Eric Harris and Dylan Klebold had killed twelve students at Columbine High School in Littleton, Colorado. Alex was asleep. As his chest rose and fell, I stared numbly at the television screens. The video clip of the students fleeing the school ran over and over again.

The ambulance arrived at eleven P.M., nearly twelve hours after Alex had been admitted to the emergency room.

It was after midnight when we arrived at Four Winds. Alex was interviewed briefly by the psychiatrist on call, and so were we. He was taken to his quarters, a rambling, two-story cottagelike building called the Lodge, where we put him to bed. We got home at three A.M. We fell into bed a few minutes later.

I woke up three hours later, without an alarm, and went to work. In midafternoon, I left work and took the train to Katonah, where Liz met me. We drove the three and a half miles from the train station to Four Winds, where we met the therapist who had been assigned to Alex. He told us that Alex had spent much of the day in bed, apparently unable to shake off the drowsiness produced by the previous night's sedation. The therapist had talked to him twice, and Alex had responded, though he hadn't been entirely forthcoming. The therapist asked to speak to Liz and me. We told him we had very different approaches to parenting, that we often argued as a result, and that we were having marital difficulties. Liz insisted on a family session with Alex, and the therapist agreed to stay late to provide it.

The three of us met at seven o'clock that evening for forty-five minutes. For the first time, Alex talked about his illness. He knew he was behaving badly at school and at home, and he wanted to think it was because he was a bad kid, not a sick kid. Why? Because "bad" was an attribute that he could change. He would rather be bad than sick, because that wasn't something he could do anything about, he told the therapist. His experience had proved that to him. Despite all his efforts, he was back in the hospital again.

Besides, being bad had fewer consequences. He had friends who behaved badly, and they didn't face serious consequences, not like going to the hospital. While he seemed to understand that he had a real illness, he still felt that if he behaved well in the hospital he ought to be allowed to go home. He didn't fully accept that he was there for medical care, and that it wasn't enough for him to behave well; he would have to show some improvement, as assessed by the doctors. I couldn't blame him for being confused about where bad behavior ended and illness began. I was confused myself, and his therapist had no ready answer. As he talked, it was clear that whatever had been growing in him in recent weeks seemed to have drained away. He was Alex again.

The next day, I was detained at work by a meeting called to look over the pages of a special issue of *Business-Week* for which I was the editor. It was an honor to be asked to edit a special issue, an important responsibility, and this was a project I'd particularly enjoyed. (The issue was wholly devoted to a photo essay on the past century of innovation.) But the timing was bad. I was having trouble getting out of work early to get to the hospital to see Alex and talk to his doctor and therapist. I didn't arrive until seven that night, just in time to see Alex's hospital psychiatrist. She said she wanted to start Alex on a low dose of an antidepressant, along with Risperdal, an antipsychotic drug, to try to organize his thinking. Risperdal could cause children to balloon in weight, she said; it could also produce dry, cottony mouth and sometimes lead to impairment in vision. The drug was the recommendation of Psychiatrist No. 6, she said, but I'd never heard that from him. I wondered who was really in charge, the hospital psychiatrist or Psychiatrist No. 6.

Liz and I got home about nine-thirty, just as Psychiatrist No. 6 called. The plan, he explained, was to keep Alex on lithium to decrease the upward and downward emotional swings, and to add an antidepressant, Celexa, to try to "melt down" his depression. The Risperdal would help clarify his thoughts and reduce his impulsivity. It might also produce a little cognitive impairment, he said. I couldn't help but feel a spike of concern when I heard that. There was some chance, the doctor explained, that the Celexa would "flip" Alex, driving him into a manic state. That seemed to be what had happened when Psychiatrist No. 1 prescribed Zoloft, after which came the episode in which Alex had smashed the clock in his elementary school and stormed out of the building.

Psychiatrist No. 6 said that if the diagnosis of bipolar disorder was correct, the Celexa would probably trigger a similar episode, but this time Alex would be in the hospital, where he wouldn't be in a position to harm himself or anyone else. If he did not have bipolar disorder, but instead was suffering from depression without accompanying mania, then the drug would help relieve the depression. In other words, this was a way to help solidify his diagnosis. If the drug "flipped" him, he had bipolar disorder. If it didn't, we would be looking for another diagnosis. The hope, the psychiatrist said, was that Alex would be off the Risperdal within a month or so. I was puzzled by all this talk about diagnosis. I thought the diagnosis had been settled. I thought we knew that Alex had bipolar disorder.

Psychiatrist No. 6 then said he was afraid that the insurance company that administered my managed care health plan would refuse to pay for any care after Friday. The insurer had initially authorized only one day at Four Winds, surprising the crisis counselor in our local emergency room. It was generally accepted that patients with bipolar disorder need more than a day to get over a crisis, she told me. Four Winds was able to persuade the insurance company to authorize two more days. But it was unclear whether the company would pay for anything more than that. (The charge, Psychiatrist No. 6 guessed, was probably $1,300 to $1,500 per day.) "This kid really needs to stay in the hospital," he said. "The insurance company does not have Alex's interests at heart." The company might have the money argument on its side, he said, but "we have the headlines."

The Columbine massacre was still all over the newspapers and dominating the television news channels. One message of all that coverage was that it was risky to ignore a kid in crisis. But was he saying there was some link between Alex and the two shooters at Columbine? I didn't know how to take this. It was ludicrous. But it was terrifying, too.

The psychiatrist urged us to do whatever we could to put pressure on the insurance company to pay for at least ten days or, better, two weeks, which would give the hospital time to refine Alex's treatment.

Alex said very little for the first few days. Only on the fifth day did he say he felt a little better. Gradually, he began to emerge from the depression that had settled into him. The staff said that he had "flat affect," the technical term for unresponsive emotions, but he was lively and responsive when Liz and I saw him in the evenings. We would bring pizza or Chinese food and sit in the common room chatting with him, asking him how his day had gone. We avoided any serious discussion about what was happening. Partly that was because we didn't want to upset him during the hour or two that we were allowed to see him. And partly it was because neither of us knew what to say. We didn't really know what was happening.

Alex's schedule, during the weekdays, looked something like this:

7 A.M., wakeup
7:30–8, breakfast

8–8:20, a discussion of "issues and goals"

8:20–9:35, room check, to look for contraband items;
  patients read or slept

9:40–11, school

11–11:45, gym

12–1 P.M., free time

1–1:30, lunch

2–2:45, "feedback" group

3–3:45, art therapy

4–4:30, community meeting

4:30–5:30, quiet hour

6–6:30, dinner

7–8, gym, or group therapy, or relaxation group

9:15, snack

10:30, curfew

11, lights off

Sometimes during relaxation time, or in the evenings, the staff allowed the patients to watch videotapes in the common room. No movie with any suggestion of violence or drugs was allowed, of course.

Patients brought their own shampoo, soap, hairbrushes, and deodorant. No aerosol deodorant was allowed. Anything that might be dangerous was kept locked up in a closet marked SHARPS: razor blades, glass containers, mirrors, pencils, pencil or makeup sharpeners, and scissors. Doors were kept locked. Patients thought to be dangerous to themselves or others were put on a fifteen-minute watch list.

There might have been two or three dozen patients in the unit at any given time. Boys and girls were in separate wings. The patients had widely different educational and social backgrounds, and each had his or her own emotional issues to deal with. Under those circumstances, trying to teach anything of substance during "school" was a noble but unrealistic, and generally unrealized, goal. When a student became upset, the staff would try to calm him or her, but if that failed, as it often did, they administered what they called a PRN, a shot of a sedative in the hip. "PRN," short for the Latin phrase *pro re nata,* means "when the situation arises," or "as needed."

Wedged among these activities were individual visits to therapists and psychiatrists. The patients could make calls from a pay phone, but it was often busy. We were lucky to talk to Alex once a day on the phone. It was difficult for us to call him unless we knew when free time was, because the staffers were reluctant to pull a child out of an activity for a phone call. On weekends, most of the therapists and psychiatrists were away, except when there was an emergency. I came to think of weekend days in the hospital as days wasted. My insurance policy allotted the children, over their lifetimes, a total of ninety days each in psychiatric hospitals. These weekend days were eating up the insurance allotment, but doing little for Alex.

Alex told his therapist that he felt left out, especially from his family. He said his parents didn't love him, and that he was a bad person. Although he was clearly depressed, he denied that he had suicidal thoughts. He cagily admitted that maybe he had had some of those thoughts recently, but said he had no specific plans to do anything about them. And his friends had worked to talk him out of taking any action, he said. After we met with Alex and his therapist twice, the therapist concluded that Alex was deeply disturbed about the arguments between his mother and me, and that his depression was a strategy he used to defend himself against parental conflict. The therapist strongly recommended that we enter family therapy after Alex's discharge.

Alex continued a modest improvement. For the first time, he began to talk about his "disorder," admitting, to himself and to us, that he had an illness. It was an important step. The hospital confirmed the diagnosis of bipolar disorder.

For the first time, I started to read about bipolar disorder. Somebody told me about *An Unquiet Mind,* by Kay Redfield Jamison, a professor of psychiatry at Johns Hopkins School of Medicine. The book tells the story of her own experiences with bipolar disorder, which had nearly led her to suicide on more than one occasion. In evocative and elegiac prose, Jamison paints a picture of a horrible, frightening disease. Midway through the book, her condition is so desperate that it is nearly impossible to believe that she could have survived to write her memoir. By the end, she has not only survived, but has embraced the illness as a vital part of who she is. *An Unquiet Mind* helped me understand bipolar disorder, but, more than that, it gave me hope that Alex, too, might survive this thing, and might be a better man for having gone through it.

This simple act of picking up a book and deciding to learn more about Alex's condition was an important step for me. For the first time, I admitted to myself that Alex's illness was not going to magically disappear, that he wasn't going to grow out of it. I abandoned, finally, the idea that we would pull together and get through this.

Because Alex was adept at following the hospital's rules for behavior, he was transferred to another unit, in a separate building, where he had a little more privacy, a little more freedom, and the chance to play video games. It was a reward for good behavior. A day later, he was pronounced "significantly improved," with a stable mood and a good understanding of his need for treatment. This sudden improvement came on the day that he exhausted his insurance coverage. He was pronounced well enough to go home. Liz and I were told to be open about our "significant marital conflicts," and urged, again, to seek family therapy.

I didn't see Alex the day he was released. I was driving Matt, Alicia, and a friend of Alicia's to Ann Arbor, Michigan, so that Matt could take one more look at the University of Michigan before he began as a freshman the following September. Alex had a shaky weekend. He might have been "significantly improved," but he hadn't entirely healed. He had friends over to the house for a barbecue on the weekend, and Liz was able to spend a lot of time with him while the rest of us were away. Matt, Alicia, and I returned on the Sunday following Alex's discharge. We hadn't been home more than a couple of hours when the phone rang. It was the police. Alex and a friend had been picked up for trespassing on the railroad tracks. Four days or so out of the hospital, and Alex was at the police station. Again.

We picked him up at the station. I didn't let him say a word. Every time he opened his mouth, I yelled at him to close it. I told him how angry I was. I tried to explain the twin perils he faced: running afoul of the law, and putting himself in danger. He was not in any shape to listen or to have a constructive conversation. Neither was I, although I couldn't stop myself from yelling at him. Alex had learned to use the discord between Liz and me. He played us against one another, talking to one and shunning the other. At that time, Liz was the favored parent. She talked to him when we got home. I gave up and went to bed.

When Alex returned to school, he discovered that he had a new reputation. He had been picked up by the police on April 20, which was not only the day of the Columbine massacre, but a date celebrated by many marijuana users as National Pot Smokers' Day. The students at George Washington Middle School had decided that Alex must have been picked up by the police for possession. Soon Alex found himself unwelcome in homes all over Ridgewood. At the time, I did not know any of this was happening. I'd never heard of National Pot Smokers' Day, so of course I had no idea that it was familiar to middle-school kids in Ridgewood. I don't know whether any of Alex's classmates observed the occasion by smoking marijuana, but, as far as I knew, there hadn't been any arrests. Or none that had been made public. (That was an important caveat in Ridgewood. Drug arrests, sexual assaults, and other distasteful and criminal incidents often didn't make the papers.) I remembered taking Alex to visit one of his friends, who, Alex told me, was not allowed to have Alex in the house. Alex didn't tell me why, and I guessed it was because the parents knew about Alex's illness, and didn't want him socializing with their son. It wasn't until years later, when I was working on this book, that Alex told me that he'd been tagged all over Ridgewood as a druggie. He didn't tell his therapist at the time, either. It was a burden that he bore alone.

Toward the end of that school year, Alex and I had a titanic argument. The memory haunts me. I was coming home from work one evening when I ran into Alicia, around the corner from the house. "Wait until you see Alex's hair," she said. He had been talking about bleaching it blond, and I had told him he could not do that. At the time, there were plenty of boys on MTV with bleached heads, but not too many in Ridgewood. I didn't want Alex to be a pioneer in this particular fashion. I think I was afraid that it would call attention to him, as, once again, the kid who was different.

My anger built as I rounded the corner and walked toward the house. I began to lose control even before I saw him. I walked in the back door, dropped my briefcase on a chair, and went out to the front of the house, where, Alicia had told me, Alex was playing catch with a friend. I saw him at the end of the street. "Alex, get in the house right now!" I yelled. "I want to talk to you." He was far enough away that I couldn't make out exactly how his hair looked, but as he got closer, I shuddered. He smiled nervously when I called to him, but the smile faded as he came closer. "When did this happen?" I said. He told me he'd done it that afternoon, when he got home from school. A friend had come over to help him. I followed him in the house and began to scream at him. He was grounded, I told him, for I didn't know how long. He would have to have his hair dyed back to its natural color at a hairstyling salon, and he would have to use his own money to do it, even though that would probably consume most of his small savings account. I didn't stop yelling until he was in tears. I remember him saying, "I want to go to a good college." We were all excited about Matt's acceptance to the University of Michigan. My attack had so shattered Alex that he felt the incident with his hair was one more piece of evidence that he wasn't good enough to get into college, like Matt. A few days later, he had his hair dyed back to its natural sandy brown.

A few months after that, he asked permission to bleach his hair again. I shrugged and said okay. The next day, he was blond again. And it looked good on him. In one of my favorite pictures of Alex, his hair is bleached; he's crossed his arms and he's flashing a huge grin at the camera. Why had I become so angry when he had bleached it the first time? It had been a devastating blow to his sense of worth. The only answer I've come up with is that my anger was a manifestation of my own concerns about Alex, about whether he would be marked as a kid who was different. I didn't want him to be different, and I didn't want him to look different.

But the damage had been done. I asked Alex, long afterward, whether he knew why I had been so angry. "I have no idea," he said.

"I don't know, either," I told him. "I'm sorry."

have been a journalist for twenty years. During that time, I have written thousands of stories about medicine, climate change, agriculture, outer space, the tobacco industry, drugs, genetics, and other scientific and environmental issues. But, until I started work on this book, I had rarely written about psychiatry, a field in which speculation and hypothesis seemed to overshadow scientific understanding. I've been interested in the harder sciences—astronomy, chemistry, and physics, especially—as far back as I can remember. When I was five or six, my mother would stop at the library on the way home from work and bring me a stack of astronomy books, or kids' books on engineering or on the space program. I started subscribing to *Scientific American* in grade school, and by the time I was a senior in high school, I was able to persuade the physics teacher and the principal to let me skip class and just show up for the tests, because I already knew more than I would learn in the course. I got an A in the class, and went on to study physics at MIT, where I received a bachelor's degree and then decided, after all those years, that I didn't want to become a scientist after all. But that rigorous scientific background has remained with me. As friends and family often remind me, I can be maddeningly rational at times when I should show a little compassion and understanding.

All this is part of the reason I'd been dubious about psychiatry. Very little is known about the causes of psychiatric illnesses or about the drugs used to treat them. Tens of millions of Americans have taken Prozac or one of the other newer, similar antidepressants, yet researchers still do not know exactly how these drugs work, or why, in some people, they don't work at all. The principal drugs used to treat bipolar disorder, lithium and Depakote, were discovered by accident when doctors gave them to patients for other reasons, and then observed that some patients with stormy moods seemed to feel better. All branches of medicine are a mix of art and science, but in psychiatry, there is little science, and lots of art.

I'd started out as a general assignment newspaper reporter, covering cops, courts, and city hall. Editors who knew that I had a scientific background assigned me to cover science stories, energy shortages, environmental disasters, and nuclear power, and I eventually developed expertise in a broad range of sciences, far beyond what I'd learned at MIT. Yet nothing I had learned as a writer was helping me understand why Alex was behaving as he was. If I started writing about psychiatry, I thought, I would develop some expertise there, too, and I might discover something that would help my son. I'd also be making contacts with the nation's leading psychiatrists and researchers. Instead of using my work to escape from what was going on at home, I decided I had no choice but to use my professional opportunities to try to help Alex. It was time for me to put aside the prejudices about psychiatry that I had grown up with, to open my mind, and to learn something.

In the spring of 1999, when Alex was in eighth grade, I was due in Washington for a meeting. I decided to go a day early to talk to someone at the National Institute of Mental

Health, in Bethesda, Maryland. I made an appointment with Dr. Peter Jensen, who was then the director of child and adolescent psychiatry at NIMH. (He has since moved to Columbia University in New York.) I was nervously fumbling with my notebook when I walked into Jensen's office. I wanted to write something about mental illness in kids, I told him, but I had another reason for being there: my son had bipolar disorder, and I wanted to learn more about it. This was the first time I had gone into an interview admitting I had a personal stake in a story. Jensen might well have asked me to leave. I had made the appointment under false pretenses. While he might make time for a reporter, he couldn't make time for every bewildered parent who wanted to talk to him, and that's just what I was.

But Jensen didn't ask me to leave; instead, he spent two hours talking to me about the kinds of disorders that afflict children, what's known about them, and what can be done. Two or three decades earlier, he explained, doctors had believed that a newborn child was a blank tablet on which parents then proceeded to write an emotional and intellectual story. "The idea was they would be fine if the parents behaved okay," Jensen said. "That idea permeated child psychiatry. It overvalued the influence of the environment on a child, and it undervalued the things we don't know about, the things going on inside."

Children, he told me, can suffer from many of the same disorders that afflict adults, including anxiety, posttraumatic stress disorder, and depression. But children are more difficult to diagnose. "The diagnostic terms are slippery," Jensen said. "It's hard to know what they refer to in the brain." Drugmakers are reluctant to test drugs in children, fearing that they would be liable if something went wrong. And desperate parents don't want to enroll their children in studies in which the kids might get a placebo. "They want their kids to stay on drugs that seem to be helping," Jensen said. As a consequence, few of the drugs approved for treatment of mental illness in adults (Alex had now taken a number of them) have been tested in children.

I'd worried about what these drugs might be doing to Alex. Jensen told me I wasn't alone. "I don't see too many parents choosing lightly to put their children on psychiatric medications," he said. "It's usually an agonizing decision, as you know." Jensen and others have tried to encourage testing of psychiatric drugs in children; they've made some progress, but not nearly enough. "Kids," Jensen said, "are research orphans."

Most of the psychiatric drugs given to children have never been tested on children. Before drugs can be marketed and sold, their makers need to show, through costly experiments, that the drugs are both safe and effective. Those studies, routinely done on adults, earn the drugs approval from the U.S. Food and Drug Administration. At that point, the drugs go on sale, and the drug companies have little incentive to do any further testing in children. Under the FDA's regulations, doctors can prescribe any drug, once it has been approved, to anyone, including a child. The rationale is that once the FDA has ruled that drugs are safe and effective, it doesn't want to be in the business of telling doctors how to use them.

So the use of psychiatric drugs on Alex and other children amounts to a huge, unregulated, potentially dangerous experiment. Millions of children are getting drugs that haven't been shown to be safe and effective in children. Many of these drugs appear to be helpful, of course, and no one is suggesting that doctors stop prescribing them. The difficulty is that they may have unsuspected side effects. They might, for example, inflict subtle damage on the thinking and learning ability of young, not fully developed brains. A 1997 federal law offered drugmakers a six-month extension on their patents if they voluntarily tested their drugs on children, but this incentive was insufficient: Why perform tests, when the drugs were already being sold to children? Testing the drugs wouldn't increase sales to children, but it could decrease sales sharply if the testing found that the drugs were unsafe for children. In 1998, the FDA enacted a regulation called the pediatric rule, under which it could require the testing of drugs in children. Antiregulatory groups challenged the rule, on the grounds that it would raise the cost of drug approvals. A court struck down the rule. The result is that drug companies save the extra money it would have taken to test drugs in children. And the experimental, untested use of the drugs continues. Psychiatrists are faced with a dilemma: Use the untested drugs in children, or offer them no medication at all.

This is not merely a theoretical concern. Problems do arise. In early June 2003, British drug regulators reviewed nine studies of Paxil, a widely prescribed antidepressant, and concluded that it raised the risk of suicide in children. The regulators said that Paxil (known as Seroxat in Britain) should not be given to children. "It has become clear that the benefits of Seroxat in children for the treatment of depressive illness do not outweigh these risks," the regulators said. A week or so later, the FDA said that no one under eighteen should be given Paxil. Neither the FDA nor the British regulatory agency reached definitive conclusions about the safety of the drug, which is part of the class of newer antidepressants that includes Prozac and Zoloft. But the lack of a definitive conclusion was precisely the problem: The studies that could be done to answer the safety question definitively were not done. The drug's manufacturer, GlaxoSmithKline, refused to take a position. "It's difficult for me sitting here to tell doctors what they should do with their patients," a company executive said.

Paxil was then Glaxo's best-selling drug. In October 2003, the FDA said it had reviewed all the evidence and could not determine whether Paxil and other similar antidepressants, such as Zoloft, Celexa, and Prozac, increased the risk of suicide in children and adolescents. British regulators, however, came to a radically different conclusion. By December, they had become so alarmed about the possibility of increased suicide risk that they told doctors not to prescribe any of these antidepressants to children or teenagers—except for Prozac.

Some experts expressed skepticism about the concern, saying that the drugs, by effectively treating depression in children, had undoubtedly prevented many suicides. Any risk that the drugs might trigger suicide was likely to be outweighed by the suicides they prevented, these authorities said. For the parents of mentally ill children, the debate was far more than academic. They have to make the decision every day whether to seek psychiatric drugs for their children or to continue giving the drugs to children who are already taking them. The obvious advice would be for parents to check with their children's psychiatrists and therapists. But a psychiatrist's or therapist's decision can be based only on a hunch or a supposition or some vague feeling, because psychiatrists and therapists don't know whether the drugs are safe for children or not. No one does.

The consequences of the spectacular failure of the health care system to provide for mentally ill children can be devastating. Emotional and behavioral disorders do more than any other illness to lower quality of life and diminish educational and career opportunities for children. "No other set of conditions is close in the magnitude of its deleterious effects on children and youth," says Dr. David R. Offord of McMaster University in Hamilton, Ontario. Children with mental illness are at high risk of dropping out of school, and even if they are fortunate enough to receive treatment, they face a long and steep road back toward assuming adult responsibilities, finding work, and raising families.

A month after I saw Jensen, the American Psychiatric Association held its annual meeting in Washington, and I made plans to attend. A few days before I left, I told Alex I would be away at a psychiatrists' meeting. "I'm thinking of writing a book on mental illness in children," I told him.

"Would I be in it?" he asked.

"Yes," I said, "if that's okay with you."

He smiled. I thought, I hoped, that he took it as an expression of the depth of my concern for him. I'd just given him a copy of Kay Redfield Jamison's memoir, the first book that I had read on bipolar disorder. He'd managed to get through the first couple of chapters. In it, Jamison describes the scorching depression and uncontrolled mania that led her to the brink of suicide. It was a revelation to Alex that somebody else had gone through this. I told him Jamison would be at the meeting. He asked whether I could have her sign his book, and I told him I would try. Later, at the meeting, I caught Jamison at a dinner seminar, and interrupted her in the middle of her meal. "My son has bipolar disorder, and he's reading your book," I sputtered. "Could you sign a copy for him?" She put down her fork.

"How old is he?" she asked. I told her he was fourteen. "That's tough," she said. I handed her a copy of the book and a pen. She signed her name and wrote, "To Alex: Things will get better." Alex smiled when he saw it. "Thanks," he said.

For three weeks after he got out of the hospital, Alex attended a day treatment program a short bus ride away from home. The doctors at the hospital had recommended it as a way for Alex to ease back into school and a regular routine. Such programs are often used for just this purpose. The day was broken down into a group therapy session, private therapy, and school. The program was supposed to be, in part, a substitute for school, but the circumstances made any real teaching almost impossible. Students came and went unpredictably, as their conditions worsened or improved, or their insurance ran out. It was unclear to me whether the program was helping him much emotionally, and easy to see that it was doing nothing for him academically. He was falling further and further behind. His behavior, however, was exemplary. He was focused and able to concentrate on his work. He completed his assignments and asked for help when he needed it. The program's officials recommended that he return to his regular school.

Alex's moods slowly leveled out over the last two months of that school year. But keeping himself steady took all of his energy. As after his first hospitalization, he was unable to recover academically. In the hospital, in the special school during sixth grade, and in the day treatment program, he'd progressed wonderfully. As soon as he returned to the regular school, however, his entire personality seemed to change. His reading and writing skills were still above grade level. But he was easily distracted and had trouble completing his assignments. Frustration overwhelmed him.

Nothing seemed to help. Gradually, he abandoned schoolwork altogether. In the months after his release from the hospital, he never could catch up. Perhaps fueled by boredom, he fell back into being disruptive in class. He was flippant with teachers. When he was assigned detention, he skipped it. He was suspended after disrupting an eighth-grade assembly in early June. In utter desperation, the school principal finally told him not to show up for the rest of the school year. Alex received no home schooling, no tutoring, nothing. The principal assured Alex that he would be graduated from the eighth grade and move on to high school, but there was considerable doubt about whether he would be allowed to participate in the graduation ceremony. The principal was concerned that Alex wouldn't behave with decorum. Eventually, he relented. Alex behaved well, and the school year was over. It was a ragged ending to a difficult year.

It was difficult for me to understand how Alex could miss so much schoolwork and still move up to high school. I asked his teachers and his counselor, but I never received a clear explanation. I have always suspected that the answer had something to do with the unwillingness of Ridgewood's institutions to deal with these problems directly. If they couldn't send Alex to a private school outside the district, then they wanted to move him through the system and get him out the door. I'm not sure I would have preferred the alternative; it would have devastated Alex to be held back in the eighth grade. But Ridgewood High School was academically demanding. How would Alex manage without proper preparation?

Ridgewood High School sends almost all its graduates to college and has limited patience for students who struggle. Liz and I were not sure that Alex belonged there. We looked at a private school in town that seemed as though it might be a better fit for him. The classes were small, the teachers supportive, and the school day ended in time for Alex to make football practice at Ridgewood High School, which was a few blocks away. He'd played football for several years already, although his young career had frequently been interrupted by injuries. The previous year, he had missed the entire season after a tackle during preseason practice in which he was forced backward while his feet went forward. Amid the clatter of helmets, pads, and spikes, everyone on the field could hear the loud crack as Alex's right foot broke during the fall. He sat on the sidelines all season with his foot in a cast. He was eager to play, and the high school assured us that he would be welcome to participate in sports, even if he was going to school somewhere else.

That wasn't enough for Alex. He was heartbroken at the thought of not attending Ridgewood High School. He wanted so badly to be "normal," as he said over and over again, and he thought that the move to high school was a chance to start fresh. The previous June, Alex had attended Matt's graduation from the public high school. Matt had done well: He got good grades, ran track and cross-country for four years, was a member of the National Honor Society, and created his own show in the school's television studio. Called *Sound Barrier*, it was a mix of music reviews and political commentary, and it aired on the local-access cable channel.

The graduation ceremony was held on a warm, sunny day on the green grass of the football field. The boys wore rented white tuxedo jackets and black pants, with red boutonnieres. The girls wore white dresses and carried red bouquets. It was a happy day. One by one, the graduates were called to the front to receive their diplomas, as their parents, gathered in the football stands, took pictures. Liz and I were midway up the stands; Alex stood below us, in the first row, watching quietly, wearing his Walkman. I don't know what he was thinking, but he must have been wondering whether he would one day stand out on the field with a white jacket and boutonniere. I was wondering, too.

In the days after Matt's graduation, we continued to look for a school for Alex, and Alex continued to press the case for Ridgewood High. The truth was, I wasn't enthusiastic about the alternative schools we'd looked at, except for the one he'd attended in sixth grade, which also had a high school program. But Alex refused to go back there. In mid-July, he was tested again by the school psychologist, who found "unresolved emotional issues, including depressed mood and a high level of anxiety." As part of the testing, Alex was shown a picture of a boy contemplating a violin on a table in front of him, and was asked to explain what was happening. "This boy is being made to play the violin by his parents," Alex said. "He hates to play. He feels annoyed and sad. He'll end up smashing the violin. He used to obey his parents but he's tired of it." The psychologist concluded that Alex would be able to "function adequately" at Ridgewood High School. Alex pleaded with us to let him go to school with his old classmates. We relented.

At the end of June, Liz and I were at a party in the neighborhood when we got a call from Alicia, who was at home. She said the police had called asking about our son, and they wanted a call back. I wasn't sure which son they were talking about. Alicia didn't know, either. We went home and called. It was Alex. He'd been picked up in a bank parking lot in downtown Ridgewood with a group of seven or so kids, some of whom had alcohol and marijuana. One of the officers volunteered to bring him home. About fifteen minutes later she showed up at the door with Alex. He had not had alcohol or marijuana on him, she explained, but merely being with kids who had them was itself a violation. Alex could have been charged with possession. But he had been cooperative, she explained, so no charges were filed. Two of the other kids had been charged with possession of alcohol and drugs.

While the officer was explaining the business about access to drugs being a violation, Alex started to say something that struck me as flip, and I cut him off: "Don't start with that attitude of yours tonight." The officer finished what she was saying and left. Alex said he wanted to talk. He and Liz and I sat down around the dining room table. He hadn't been taking an attitude with me, he said. He had wanted to explain something. I looked down at the table for a moment, wondering why I had jumped on him so quickly. I told him I was sorry. He said he had tried alcohol and marijuana, but that he knew he shouldn't be messing around with them. This hadn't been his fault tonight, he said. He didn't have any of the beer or pot that several of the other kids had brought with them. Fine, I said, I'm glad you weren't charged with possession. But he didn't seem to get that being in a group of other kids who had drugs or beer could get him in trouble. Still angry, I tried to explain that he shouldn't be spending time with those kids if they were going to get him in trouble. Alex got angry in return, because I wasn't giving him credit for keeping away from the beer and drugs. "You hate me!" he yelled. "You don't care about me the way my friends do." He said he had to use the phone, and I told him he couldn't. "It's my house, and it's my phone, and you're not calling your friends!" I shouted. "You can call your friends in the morning. Now you can go up to your room and go to bed. The night is over." We continued to yell at each other, until he stopped, sat down at the table again, starting to hyperventilate. He was breathing very heavily and noisily, looking as though he were about to explode. "I have to call my friends," he kept saying. "I have to call my friends. I have to call my friends. . . ."

"Look at you," I said, "you're acting crazy." As soon as the words were out of my mouth, I wanted to take them back. He was furious. You think I'm crazy, don't you? he shouted. You don't care about me. Tears streamed down his

face. No, I said, no, I don't think you're crazy. You're just acting like you're crazy, but you're not crazy. You have to settle
down.

I regained some control over myself. But I knew I had
done it again. I had lost control and said something that Alex,
and I, would remember for a long time. I seemed to have no
ability to anticipate the consequences of my anger until the
instant I had done something unforgivable. I'm not up to this
job, I thought. I don't know how to raise my own son. I don't
know how to cope with his illness. I don't even know
whether I can get my head together enough to understand
the implications of what I'm saying before I say it. Things
move too quickly for me. I can't think ahead enough, in real
time, to come up with the right answers. I just keep coming
up with the wrong ones.

Alex and I kept talking. He calmed down. I was sorry I'd
told him he couldn't talk to his friends. He'd tried to do the
right thing in difficult circumstances, and I was punishing
him. I'd learned that he responded to the limits that had been
set in the hospital and the private school he'd attended. I was
trying to figure out how to do that at home, too, but it was
coming out all wrong. This was the wrong time to set limits,
I thought, and these were the wrong limits. Or should I stick
with what I'd done? I told him he could call his friends. I
reached up to hug him. He was an inch or two taller than
me. "I love you," I said. Tears were rolling down his face, and
mine, too. He said he wouldn't use alcohol or drugs, and that
he would give up smoking, a habit he'd acquired in the previous couple of years. That's good, I said.

Alex began his freshman year at Ridgewood High School
after Labor Day. By the end of September, he was already fal-

tering. He had started football practice, which he loved. The harder the coach worked him on the field, the more he liked it. After the first couple of weeks of practice, when the players got their uniforms, pads, and helmets, it turned out that all of the kids were able to suit up but one. There must have been a hundred kids trying out for freshman football, and Alex was the only one who didn't have a helmet. His head was too big, the coach told him. They didn't have a helmet that size. I offered to buy one at the local sports store, but the coach said that wasn't possible; all the helmets had to be approved and purchased by the school.

Alex watched from the sidelines for several days as the other kids began scrimmaging, blocking, and tackling. By the end of the week, he'd quit. How could he conclude anything other than that he wasn't wanted on the team? And, besides, his head was too big. Intentionally or not, the coach was sending Alex a powerful message: You don't "fit." I couldn't understand this. Alex was a big kid, but he wasn't any bigger than most of the rest of them. And yet he was the only one who didn't have a helmet. I went to see the coach Saturday morning at the beginning of practice, promising myself that I would control my anger so that I didn't embarrass Alex. I found the coach lounging over a chair, all arms, legs, and muscles, bantering with a couple of other coaches. The place smelled like wintergreen mixed with the rubbery scent of new sneakers. These guys were everything I am not, with their raspy voices, ruined from years of shouting at their players; their lumpy, muscled arms and legs; their over-size sweatshirts with the sleeves torn off. I was nearly in tears. I asked for an explanation.

"We don't have a helmet now that fits him," the coach bellowed. "Should be arriving soon."

"That's not good enough," I stammered. "He thinks you

don't want him on the team, and I think he's right. That's exactly the message you are sending him." I asked the coach to come over to our house later that day and explain to Alex that he shouldn't take this personally, that he'd be out on the field in a few days. The coach grudgingly agreed. Later that afternoon, he showed up at the house and told Alex that he wanted him back on the team as soon as the helmets arrived. He didn't stay long, and Alex barely spoke. When the coach left, Alex was furious at me. I had embarrassed him by asking the coach to come to the house. It was Alex's last experience with school sports. A gifted natural athlete, he never tried out for a team again.

Perhaps there was more to it. In *An Unquiet Mind,* Jamison talks about how the side effects of taking lithium had kept her from playing squash and even riding horses. "Sports were fun only up to a point," she wrote. "Lithium threw off my coordination." She had to give up riding because she kept falling off the horses. She missed sports. Giving them up felt like a kind of premature aging. "Each time I had to give up a sport, I had to give up not only the fun of that sport, but also that part of myself that I had known as an athlete." Maybe the same sort of things were happening to Alex. I couldn't tell, and he wouldn't say. The lithium had given him a pronounced tremor, which made it difficult for him to write legibly. Maybe it was throwing off his coordination, too.

Or maybe the coach had some agenda. Maybe he had heard about Alex, and about the problems Alex had caused in the eighth grade, and maybe he didn't want this problem on the team. He certainly wouldn't have said so; I'm sure it would have been illegal to discriminate like that. But I couldn't pursue the matter any further. Alex was extremely sensitive about the issue, and he didn't want to talk about it. It was already too late.

In September, just after Alex began the year at Ridgewood High School, I went to the Carter Center in Atlanta. I'd been awarded one of the center's fellowships in mental health journalism. The fellowships were an outgrowth of Rosalynn Carter's long interest in mental health. I'd applied in the spring, hoping to get some support for my proposed book on mental illness in children. I planned to use the fellowship as an opportunity to get started on the book proposal. My editors at *BusinessWeek* were not enthusiastic about the prospects for writing about mental illness in the magazine, and it was with reluctance that they agreed to let me use several days of vacation time to attend a meeting of the fellows at the Carter Center.

At the Carter Center, I was required to present my project to a group consisting of about fifteen fellows, a board of distinguished psychiatrists, psychologists, and others who oversaw the program, and Rosalynn Carter. I was shaking as I stepped up to the podium. I had never talked about Alex's illness in public. I'd rarely discussed it even with friends and family. I'd left even my parents mostly in the dark. When Alex was first hospitalized, I told Liz to say that he had the flu. I hadn't wanted anyone to know that he suffered from a psychiatric ailment, and now I was about to discuss that very ailment with strangers.

It was the most sympathetic audience imaginable; these were mental health professionals and colleagues interested in mental illness. And many of them, like me, had seen it up close. Still, when I spoke, my voice quavered. I paused several times to collect myself. Somehow, I managed to get through a twenty-minute presentation. Afterward, I felt a monstrous sense of relief. Nervous energy poured out of me like spring snowmelt. It was the first time I had broken through my own fears and prejudices and begun to talk about what was happening. That was probably the single most important thing the fellowship did for me. I was leaving behind the shock, numbness, and fear with which I'd greeted Alex's illness, and I was admitting that I needed to know more.

One of the members of the board, Dr. Paul Fink, a distinguished psychiatrist and past president of the American Psychiatric Association, came up to me later. Each of the fellows had been assigned an adviser on the board. Fink was mine. "How is your son sleeping?" he asked me. Not well, I said; he's up all hours of the night, and he has a hard time waking up in the morning. Fink asked me a few more questions, and then said something I couldn't quite believe: "He's not being properly treated." Alex's lithium level wasn't high enough, Fink went on. I'd told him enough for him to feel certain that Alex's case was not being handled properly. Would I like him to intervene? Fink described the problems one of his own kids had faced. I would have to act as aggressively as possible if I wanted Alex to get proper treatment: "Your vigilance is critical," he said. He told me to think it over. If I wanted him to make a call on my behalf, to a psychiatrist friend in New York who could review Alex's case and find him better treatment, he would. Think about it, he said. And that night, at dinner, he asked me whether I'd thought about it. Make the call, I said. I want Alex to get help.

One of the books I'd picked up before the Carter Center meeting was *Lost Boys*, by James Garbarino, a Cornell

University psychologist. Garbarino, whom I'd heard speak at a scientific meeting, had spent much of his career interviewing boys who had killed someone, or tried to. I had developed a nearly obsessive interest in the shootings at Columbine High School. I clipped stories about it and other school shootings from newspapers and magazines, and I thought about writing something on the case. At the psychiatrists' meeting, I went to a session on school violence.

As Garbarino noted, the school year that ended in June 1998 had been notable for violence. On October 1, 1997, sixteen-year-old Luke Woodham killed his mother, then went to his Mississippi high school and opened fire, killing three and wounding seven. On December 1, in West Paducah, Kentucky, Michael Carneal shot and killed three students during a prayer meeting. On March 24, 1998, in Jonesboro, Arkansas, Mitchell Johnson, who was thirteen, and Andrew Golden, eleven, shot and killed four students and a teacher. On April 24, in Edinboro, Pennsylvania, Andrew Wurst, fourteen, shot and killed a teacher at a school dance. In Springfield, Oregon, May 21, Kip Kinkel shot twenty-four students, killing two. Just before he'd left for school, he'd killed his parents. Those killings were followed, not quite a year later, by the massacre at Columbine.

Most of the press coverage focused on the parents of the victims, but I kept thinking about the parents of the kids who'd fired the guns. What were they going through? Their children were killers. Could a sane child do what these children had done? The parents must be agonizing over what they'd done wrong, or failed to do right. Had they mistreated their children? Had they been decent parents who'd done their best and tragically failed? Maybe parenting had little or nothing to do with it. Maybe each of these kids would have come to that moment, with a trembling finger on a cold trigger, no matter what his parents had done. All I could think about was a growing awareness that I had failed Alex, and that my shortcomings had done something irrevocable to him.

Garbarino found that boys who kill are "in some ways like my own teenage son, yet in other ways so alien." Were they, in some ways, like my teenage son, too? Alex had threatened me, and he'd threatened Liz. He'd talked about hurting himself. Some of the boys Garbarino talked to were deeply troubled and in pain. "I came to see their toughness as a survival strategy," he wrote. "Young or old, they often seem naïve and childlike as they talk about their life." Others had "gotten lost through unfortunate accidents of human developments. . . . Adults in their lives made ordinary efforts to teach them how to live in society, but these ordinary efforts were not enough." Whether these boys deserved treatment or punishment for what they'd done, I didn't know. But what troubled me was that many of them might have easily turned out differently. They'd made choices, or faced situations, that could have gone either way. They had gotten lost, as Garbarino put it, on the way to becoming men.

I never believed that Alex could find himself in such dire circumstances; it was too fantastic and improbable. But I worried that his threats might lead to actual violence. I talked about this fear at the Carter Center, and it was a great relief to me when Fink, and some of the others, assured me that my worries were unfounded. In popular culture, mental illness and violence are closely linked. Scores of movies and books use mental illness as the "explanation" for senseless violence. Studies have shown, however, that people with mental illnesses are no more likely to be violent than anyone else. It was unlikely that Alex would become violent, Fink told me. He himself had worked with troubled kids, and he seemed to know what he was talking about. I didn't realize how frightened I'd been until his words relieved me of that burden. I exhaled, beginning to let go of some of the worries that had bothered me since I'd first seen the footage of the students at Columbine fleeing their school. Midway through Garbarino's book, I put it back on the shelf. I no longer needed to finish it.

But I did need to find out more about bipolar disorder. Jamison's book had given me considerable insight into what it was like to have the illness, but I didn't know what, if anything, was known about its causes, about the course it was likely to take, or, more specifically, what the long-term outcome might be for Alex. For a long time, I hadn't wanted to know. I'd been too afraid. Now I was beginning to feel that I needed to know. Wandering through a college bookstore on a business trip, I found a book called *Bipolar Disorder* by Francis Mark Mondimore, a psychiatrist who was then at the University of North Carolina and is now a colleague of Jamison's at Johns Hopkins. It was exactly what I was looking for.

Manic-depressive illness, or bipolar disorder, has been known since at least A.D. 150, when it was described by the Greek physician Aretaeus of Cappadocia, in Turkey. Aretaeus recorded and described symptoms of depression, or melancholia, in some of his patients, and mania in others. Despite the dramatic differences in these two conditions, he came to believe that they were two aspects of a single disorder. "In my opinion," he wrote, "melancholia is without any doubt the beginning and even part of the disorder called mania." That insight was lost in the intervening centuries, when madness was thought to be the work of devils, demons, and other evil forces.

"Bipolar disorder" is now the official scientific term for what was once called manic-depressive insanity. The newer term is intended to distinguish this disorder, with its upward and downward mood swings, from depression, sometimes called unipolar depression, in which all the swings are downward. "Bipolar disorder" is also thought to be less stigmatizing, less awful sounding, than "manic-depression." Jamison doesn't agree. "Patients who have suffered from the illness should have the right to choose whichever term they feel more comfortable with," she writes in *An Unquiet Mind*. "As a person and patient . . . I find the word 'bipolar' strangely and powerfully offensive: it seems to me to obscure and minimize the illness it is supposed to represent. The description 'manic-depressive,' on the other hand, seems to capture both the nature and the seriousness of the disease I have."

The first scientific description of manic-depression came from the German psychiatrist Emil Kraepelin, in the sixth edition of his influential *Textbook of Psychiatry*, published in 1899. Kraepelin studied the wide range of illnesses variously known as periodic and circular insanity, simple mania, melancholia, and confusional or delirious insanity, along with other morbid colorings of mood, as he called them, and wrapped them into one well-defined clinical picture: manic-depressive insanity. These various conditions "pass over one into the other without recognizable boundaries," Kraepelin wrote. The illness that comprised them was among the most common disorders among patients in his hospital, but almost unknown in children. Most of the cases he observed occurred in patients in their twenties and thirties. It appeared less often in older people and rarely in anyone under twenty.

(Not until the 1990s, almost a century later, was bipolar disorder recognized in children.) Although he noted that manic-depression ran in families, Kraepelin was unable to determine what might be causing it. "About the nature of manic-depressive insanity, we are still in complete uncertainty," he wrote. "Both the frequent return of the attacks and the peculiar alternation of excitement and inhibition are complete enigmas." He also noted that mania seemed to allow creative powers to flourish, by loosening inhibitions that might otherwise constrain it.

Jamison and others have explored the curious link between bipolar disorder and creativity. The list of artists, musicians, and writers who probably had bipolar disorder is long. There is some disagreement over who belongs on that list, but among those often mentioned are Vincent van Gogh, Edgar Allan Poe, Lord Byron, Virginia Woolf, Ernest Hemingway, Sylvia Plath, Anne Sexton, and Robert Schumann. Bipolar disorder might be what drove them, alternately, to creative heights and to depression, despair, and sometimes suicide. Woolf, Plath, Hemingway, and Sexton all killed themselves. Poe died in mysterious circumstances, spending several days lapsing in and out of consciousness after being found wandering the streets of Baltimore in 1849. His life was riven with stormy relationships and violent emotions, but those same disturbing emotions might have given rise to some of his brilliantly horrific stories and indelible, musical poetry. A study of the dates of composition of Schumann's major works reveals periods of explosive creativity alternating with years of relative creative drought. A graph of these swings back and forth looks like the mood chart of a person with bipolar disorder. Jamison studied biographical information and available medical records on

British and Irish poets born during the eighteenth century, and found that more than a third of them likely suffered from bipolar disorder. Studies of distinguished living writers, composers, and artists have come to similar conclusions. Bipolar disorder is far more common among creative people than among the rest of the population.

It is also thought to be common among political leaders and business executives, although few of them are willing to admit to it. One magazine said bipolar disorder was so common among corporate executives that it ought to be called "CEO's disease."

The links among creativity, mania, and leadership raise intriguing questions about the causes of bipolar disorder. Do the remarkable features of manic-depression and creativity share a particular set of structures in the brain?

Sadly, in the hundred years since Kraepelin observed that psychiatrists were in "complete uncertainty" about the causes of bipolar disorder, little has changed. The disease is still a mystery. And so what Kraepelin said about the treatment of bipolar disorder also remains true: "A treatment according to cause of manic-depressive insanity . . . does not exist." All he knew to do was to prevent "external stimuli" as far as possible. "This indication is met by the placing of the patient in an institution," where "we shall limit the pressure of occupation as far as possible and keep all restless patients in bed." Sometimes bromides (compounds containing the element bromine, now used in photographic emulsions, dyes, and antiknock motor fuel) were prescribed to try to ward off a manic attack. If bed rest failed, patients were prescribed long baths, even through the night, if possible. Psychotherapy consisted of "quiet friendliness," to "make the patient, who in unskilled hands is dangerous and stubborn, docile and good-natured."

Researchers may not know much more about the causes of bipolar disorder than they did in Kraepelin's day, but the treatment, thankfully, has improved enormously since then. The reason? A pair of fortunate accidents. The two treatments most commonly used for bipolar disorder—lithium and Depakote—were discovered by chance when doctors tried to use them for entirely different purposes.

The story begins in the middle of the twentieth century, when psychiatry in Europe and the United States was dominated by the followers of Sigmund Freud. Other than sedatives and opiates, few drugs were available even to ease the symptoms of mental illness. Freudian psychoanalysis was the most powerful treatment tool then known, and it was widely used. By the 1950s, "nearly every prestigious psychiatry chair in the country was occupied by an analyst," the Harvard psychiatrist J. Allan Hobson writes in *Out of Its Mind,* a critique of American psychiatry. "Analysts wrote the textbooks, ran the journals, called the shots." But psychoanalysis didn't work well with all disorders. As Mondimore points out, patients with schizophrenia and bipolar disorder, in particular, received little benefit from Freudian analysis, even if they had the time and money for the requisite four or five therapy sessions per week. Doctors tried almost everything, including quinine and cod liver oil. Nothing worked.

That helped to persuade some researchers, including John F. J. Cade of the Mental Hygiene Department in Victoria, Australia, that bipolar disorder had a biological cause. He wondered whether he could find something in the urine of people with bipolar disorder that would indicate what was wrong. He tried injecting uric acid from bipolar patients into guinea pigs, to see whether it was toxic. But he was having trouble dissolving the uric acid in water to inject it. Lithium was known to help uric acid dissolve in water, so

Cade added lithium to the mix. To find out whether it was toxic, he injected it into animals. They survived, but for a brief period they "became extremely lethargic and unresponsive." He wondered what might happen if he injected lithium into bipolar patients. Would they, too, become lethargic and unresponsive? In other words, could he neutralize their mania?

In an experiment that would never be allowed today, because of the unknown nature of the risks, he gave lithium to ten patients. Cade reported the findings of this landmark study on September 3, 1949, in the *Medical Journal of Australia*. All ten patients had shown dramatic improvement. One man, "who had been in a state of chronic manic excitement for five years, restless, dirty, destructive, mischievous and interfering," improved in three weeks. He left the hospital and went back to his job. Another patient, a fifty-year-old man who had been suffering from periodic manic attacks since he was twenty, improved in two weeks. "He was practically normal—quiet, tidy, rational," Cade reported.

As Mondimore points out, this was not entirely an accident. Cade "was pursuing a biological intervention for what he believed was a biological disorder." Had he not begun to look for a toxin in the urine of his patients, he would not have stumbled on the surprising effect of lithium.

Depakote, the brand name for a substance known either as valproate or valproic acid, came along in the 1960s. Researchers were studying several new drugs they hoped would prove effective against epilepsy, but they had run into the same problem as Cade: It was not easy to dissolve these compounds in water. So the researchers turned to valproic acid, which had been previously used to dissolve other drugs. That allowed them to continue their studies of the new drugs, but now it proved difficult to determine which of the new drugs were more effective in treating epileptic seizures. It soon became clear that none of them were. It was the valproic acid that had produced improvements. There was soon interest in trying the drug with bipolar patients, but only in the 1990s was valproic acid established as a standard treatment for bipolar disorder.

These remain the two standard drugs for treatment of bipolar disorder. And researchers still do not know how or why they work.

As I was reading Mondimore, I began to call and to visit some of the leading figures in the diagnosis and treatment of bipolar disorder in children. I soon learned that a controversy had arisen about the diagnosis. For decades after Kraepelin described the illness, most psychiatrists believed it occurred only in adults, with perhaps a few very rare exceptions. In the 1990s, however, it became clear that there was a group of children whose symptoms didn't fit well into the established categories of children's psychiatric ailments. Some psychiatrists began to argue that those children, children much like Alex, were suffering from bipolar disorder. It could be as common among children as among adults, striking perhaps one in one hundred, some psychiatrists argued. But there was no consensus. Other psychiatrists said these kids had somewhat unusual cases of, say, conduct disorder, or attention-deficit/hyperactivity disorder. The American Academy of Child and Adolescent Psychiatry, which might have stepped in to settle the controversy, hasn't done so. It has no official position on the question of bipolar illness in children, partly because so many of its members disagree. Some of the psychiatrists who treated Alex clearly did not believe bipolar disorder occurred in children, and that contributed to the difficulty of getting him a correct diagnosis.

I went to see Dr. Barbara Geller, a psychiatrist at Washington University in St. Louis who has pioneered the diagnosis of bipolar disorder in children. One reason for the controversy, she said, is that children and adults with bipolar disorder have different symptoms. Adults might suffer one or two episodes of mania and depression a year, lasting days or weeks. At other times, they feel quite normal. Children are far more likely to show what psychiatrists call rapid cycling, according to Geller. "They can jump around and feel good, then crash to suicidal depressions with no apparent cause," she told me.

In Alex, I'd seen mostly depression, not the wild mania that people talk about with bipolar disorder. But I did remember one night, earlier that spring, that seemed to me to be an example of mania. I had been sitting at the piano at home, playing and singing show tunes, as I often did when I got home from work, too exhausted to do anything else. Alex often sang with me, but this night he began to sing along much more boisterously, improvising new melodies and thoroughly enjoying himself. I was delighted to see him so happy, and we played and sang until he was exhausted. Later, I realized that Alex had been not only enthusiastic but bursting with energy, and as free of inhibitions as I'd ever seen him.

After we finished singing, we went out to a nearby restaurant. Alex ordered fried calamari, his favorite dish, and carried on a vigorous, exuberant conversation. While he was waiting for his dinner to arrive, he quieted down. And then I watched as his mood slid into a deep pit. He became silent. His shoulders fell. He hunched over the table, with his eyes downcast. His head sagged until it nearly met the table. The entire transformation took less than ten minutes. When the food arrived, I left to take him home. He wasn't able to sit at the table. It was the most dramatic example I'd ever seen of a mood swing. It wasn't frightening, because I knew what was happening, but it was sad. I sensed that he, too, was sorry to have slid from the energetic mood peak where he'd stood only a few minutes before.

Many of the parents of bipolar kids don't care how the doctors resolve the controversy over its diagnosis. They know their kids are sick, and they are convinced the illness is something different from ADHD. At a psychiatrists' meeting, I met Martha Hellander, the indefatigable mother of a bipolar child and the executive director of the Child and Adolescent Bipolar Foundation, a leading parents' group. "We don't care what the doctors call it," she told me. "We're telling them, 'We observe things you don't observe, and you need to listen to us.' Debating the issue doesn't help the children."

Increasingly, psychiatrists are accepting the view that bipolar disorder occurs in children, but there are still many questions about how to treat it. By the time I had begun to learn more about bipolar disorder in children, Alex had been on lithium for more than three years, with little improvement. He had never been treated with Depakote. It didn't occur to me that there would be much difference between the two drugs. If I'd given the matter much thought, I suppose I would have concluded that Alex was one of the unfortunates with bipolar disorder who didn't respond well to treatment. But the idea that Alex might not get better was not one I wanted to pursue.

The morning after I made my presentation at the Carter Center, Fink handed me a note with a name and phone number on it. He'd called an old friend, Dr. Clarice Kestenbaum, the head of child psychiatry at Columbia University in New York. She was then the president of the American Academy of Child and Adolescent Psychiatry. She would set something up for Alex, he said.

Alex needed help quickly. While his moods had improved, his performance in high school was deteriorating. He had begun the year in mainstream classes, with some special assistance, but his grades plummeted. He wasn't doing any homework in the evenings. He said he was getting his work done in his study periods at school, but it was evident from his grades that he wasn't. He was failing almost all his courses.

As soon as I returned home from the Carter Center meeting, I called Kestenbaum. She referred me to a psychiatrist on her staff, and I set up an appointment with him. He was about to become Alex's seventh psychiatrist. Unlike any of the other psychiatrists or psychologists Alex had seen, this one asked for copies of all the records I could find from Alex's previous treatment. I gathered as much as I could and sent him a bulging FedEx package. He asked Alex and Liz and me to fill out several questionnaires. I described myself as "sociable, generally happy, and affectionate toward Alex and very interested in his activities," but "increasingly wrapped up in work and having trouble understanding his illness." Liz said she was "often very active, must be moving all the time, and wants child to respond quickly to requests." She said she would "try not to put as much pressure on child," leaving "decision-making more to child to have him learn certain consequences." She concluded with "mother very protective and loving toward child." I wrote that ours was a "hot" home, with a lot of arguments. We spoke without thinking. Liz and I argued frequently, I wrote. On a separate form, Alex wrote that he was often unhappy, and often worried about school, and about making mistakes. He said he was often upset at home.

Psychiatrist No. 7 began to taper Alex off lithium. At the same time, he started him on Depakote, gradually increasing the dose. By the middle of November, Alex was off lithium and on Depakote. And something remarkable was happening. As the balance tipped toward Depakote, his mood had begun to improve. The change was more apparent to Liz and me than to Alex, who still felt irritable at times without knowing why. He told Psychiatrist No. 7 he didn't think he would ever get better. But I had noticed a substantial change. I sent the psychiatrist an e-mail telling him that Alex's mood had improved enormously since the beginning of November. It was like flipping a switch, I said. Lithium and Depakote were the two drugs most widely used to treat bipolar disorder; I wondered why Psychiatrist No. 6 had kept him on lithium, which didn't seem to be working terribly well, instead of trying Depakote.

Alex's sleep schedule was still off, but he was sleeping less during the day and doing better at night. He seemed on track toward a regular cycle. He seemed like a new kid, a different kid, or, really, the old kid back again. Instead of letting his head droop, he held it high. He was happy. One week, Alex and I spent three evenings watching TV together, talking and joking. We hadn't had that kind of relaxed, easy interchange for a long, long time.

A few days later, he decided he wanted to learn to play the guitar. I wrote down a few chords for him to practice and bought him a beginner's guitar book, and within a few days he was banging out the chords for "Mr. Tambourine Man" well enough so that Alicia and I could sing along. We went to the piano, where I played some of the songs from *Les Misérables,* and Alex joined Alicia and me in singing along. I kept them up until after eleven. I read them a story, and we all went to bed. A happy, quiet evening at home. It was a rare thing.

CHAPTER FIVE

t is early spring, at night, the time of year when the weather is jittery and uncertain. One evening gives a premature glimpse of summer; the next is one of winter's last biting shots. On one of those evenings, Alicia is upstairs in her bedroom, alone. She takes a bottle of Tylenol out of the medicine cabinet in the upstairs bathroom. I'm sitting downstairs. It's about the time I'd be finishing dinner after a late night at work, and catching up on the magazines piled on the end of the dining room table, or idly playing the piano. Liz would be in the other room, watching television or paying the bills. Alicia counts out fifteen tablets, pours herself a glass of water, and swallows them. This takes a few minutes; she can't swallow very many at once. She goes back to her bedroom, closes the door, and turns off the lights. She slips underneath the covers and waits. She waits to fall asleep, not expecting to wake up. It is the only way she can think of to put an end to the torture she is going through at school. She is twelve years old, and in the sixth grade.

Some of the sixth-grade girls, the "popular" girls as Alicia calls them, have conspired to attack her. They've been spreading tales that she has been sexually involved with who knew how many of the boys in their class. This is not true.

Alicia was spotted kissing the boyfriend of one of the "popular" girls. That triggered the attack. By the time Alicia takes the pills, she has been enduring it for weeks. At first, some of Alicia's girlfriends helped her fend off this kangaroo court's charges. But it's difficult to sway sixth-grade girls once they have made up their minds. Most of the girls didn't believe Alicia's denials, no matter how vigorously she or her friends repeated them. Her friends began to desert her. Alicia was a "slut," everybody thought so, and who wanted to be seen with a girl like that? School became unbearable. Alicia didn't tell Liz, or me, or anyone else who might have helped her. Later she said it was because Alex's troubles seemed so much "louder" than hers. All our attention had been diverted to him.

On this night, Alicia has decided that she can't endure the attack any longer. As she's lying in bed, her stomach starts to cramp. She runs to the bathroom, where she begins throwing up violently. Liz hears her and climbs the stairs to the bathroom to help. Alicia doesn't say anything about why she's throwing up. She seems better afterward, and she's fine the next day. We decide it must be some sort of twenty-four-hour bug.

The situation at school settled down later in the spring. The attackers grew weary of that particular diversion, abandoned it, and moved on to something or someone else. Some of the girls who had deserted Alicia became her friends again. But the episode left her with a corrosive residue of pain that persisted long after the attacks ended. She became depressed. She had trouble falling asleep, and she couldn't eat. She lost what she guessed was five or ten pounds over a period of a few weeks. She had difficulty concentrating. Her schoolwork suffered. The symptoms eased during the summer, while she was away from school, but they returned almost immediately when she began the seventh grade in the fall.

Neither Liz nor I knew what was going on. While I was at the Carter Center, in September, making the contacts that would be crucial in obtaining better treatment for Alex, Alicia was slipping into a bleak landscape of her own. She seemed moody. At times, she became distant. I saw this, but I didn't worry too much about it. I thought I knew what was happening: she was becoming a teenager. And this was just what I expected, what was supposed to happen: she would gradually become more distant from her parents and closer to her friends. So I didn't question Alicia too much; I thought she needed to be left alone, to be given a little space of her own. She didn't tell us about the trouble at school, and her friends had deserted her. So she had to face the problem alone.

Taking the Tylenol ultimately hadn't produced much relief. So she decided to try something else. "I was reading a book, one of those 'teenage outcry for help' books, with all their stories about their depression," she told me a few years later. "In my case, that was not helpful at all. I thought, 'This is the way I should be feeling, because a lot more people feel like this.' And one of the things somebody wrote about was cutting. And I was like, Hey, that sounds like that might be helpful." She broke open one of her disposable razors and took out the blades. She pressed the edge of a blade against her upper arm and drew it slowly across the skin. It produced a thin stripe of blood. She watched the blood gather, form a droplet, and trickle down her arm. The sight was strangely calming, she told me later. Whatever pain she might have experienced from the cutting was overwhelmed by the sense of relief she felt when she watched herself bleed.

Alicia and I had what I thought was a nearly ideal relationship. We shared many interests. We liked each other's music. We enjoyed unusual restaurants. We would sometimes drive into New York to go to a Broadway show. We would read to each other at night, and she would write in her journal, and we would compare notes on our writing. So I had few worries about her, even as she became more distant and spent more time in her room, alone or on the telephone or listening to music. It never occurred to me that she might be depressed. And I'd never heard of children cutting themselves to get emotional relief. Perhaps she was upset by the marital strife, and seeking some shelter, I thought.

Until things began to sour for her in the sixth grade, Alicia's school experience had been like Alex's. Both children were friendly, well-liked, and socially adept. Both were bright, original, and creative. Both were quickly identified as standouts in the classroom. "You were a leader, both socially and academically," Alicia's third-grade teacher told her at the end of the year. "I will always remember you as a bright young lady who maintained high expectations for herself." This was typical of the comments Alicia received in grade school.

Alicia made friends readily and developed an easy sophistication around adults. She was a favorite of her teachers, not only because she was a good student but because she was intelligent, articulate, and comfortable around them. She spent plenty of time with her friends, but she was always eager to take a trip to a museum, or to the theater, or other more wordly settings. I occasionally took her along to events I attended in connection with my job. One night, when she was twelve, we went to a dinner at which I was covering talks by Harrison Ford and the primatologist Jane Goodall. We chatted with the two of them before the dinner, and Alicia easily joined the conversation. Before she was through, she had charmed them, too. She spent time alone talking with Goodall. We sat at different tables during the dinner (I was at the press table). After dinner, a woman who sat at Alicia's table told me Alicia had spent the evening discussing movies and had expressed a preference for independent films.

From the time she was very young, Alicia was a precocious reader. She also liked to write and tell stories. Sometimes when I read to her at night, she asked that I put down whatever book we were reading and make up a story. So we began, occasionally, to tell stories to each other at bedtime. She had a feeling for language, and a happy, unfettered imagination. Her fifth-grade teacher told us that Alicia's sophistication as a reader was "truly outstanding." At the end of the year, this teacher wrote: "She is well prepared for all of the new experiences that she will face as she moves on" to middle school.

Less than a year later, Alicia had slipped into a profound depression.

During the summer between sixth and seventh grade, Alicia began keeping a journal. That was where, for the next two and a half years, she would record her most personal thoughts. She wrote late at night, sometimes while on the phone with a friend, sometimes while listening to music by Ani DiFranco or Fiona Apple. She allowed me to look through her diaries while I was working on this book. The story they tell, in explicit, personal language, sometimes reflects what I knew was going on with Alicia. But at other points, it is wildly at odds with what I thought was happening.

To me, for instance, the summer between sixth and seventh grades seemed relatively uneventful for her. The journals tell a different story. "I'm a terrible daughter. I never do anything right. I'm crap," she wrote. "I'm depressed, but who gives a fuck. No one." Earlier one evening, her mother had yelled at her about leaving wet bath towels on the floor in her room, and dirty dishes in the sink. "Alex can do whatever he wants, no one cares. . . . Alex has gone through 'hell.' So have I! But no one takes the time to notice."

Alicia wrote that she sat on her bed and cried. Then she started rocking back and forth, saying she didn't want to be alive. "Then I stopped," she wrote. "I felt a calm like nothing I'd ever felt. My body was at peace. I was going to try to kill myself." A phone call from a friend interrupted the thought. After the call, she used her scissors to cut herself twice. "I can't live like this," she wrote. "I don't want to commit suicide because I hate myself. I want to do it because it'll cause my parents pain." Alicia went into the bathroom and took four pills from a bottle of Aleve. "Hopefully, I'll feel pain from it," she wrote. And maybe her parents would notice something was wrong: "I just want something to happen to me to make them worry the way they do about Alex."

This was what that summer was like for Alicia. From the outside, she seemed reasonably happy. Inside her head, however, she was wrestling with parents who treated her unfairly and didn't give a damn about her, and a brother who needed most of the sympathy and understanding in the family, leaving little left over for her. She was contemplating suicide and cutting herself repeatedly. She was careful to hide the wounds on her upper arms. Liz and I never spotted them.

By the fall, Alicia began to change in ways more obvious to us. She was unhappy all the time. If this was the beginnings of adolescence, she had it bad. She was listless and sad. In school, where she had always done well, she was beginning to falter. This was around the time when Alex was beginning to emerge from his darkest days. After years of denying that anything was wrong with Alex, after trying to wish it away, I had learned that I was wrong. I had learned that he was sick and needed help. And now that help was starting to pay off. He was getting better. Now, I thought, we could look forward to a less complicated family life. I was beginning to relax. I felt lighter, happier. *We were going to get through this.* And yet, despite what I'd learned from our experiences with Alex, I at first missed what was happening to Alicia. As I realized that she, too, was slipping into a profound emotional illness, I felt inept and stupid. How could I have missed this again? I was uncaring, clueless. As a father, I was a failure. I couldn't see any other way to explain it.

Alicia was in worse shape than we knew. On November 7, 1999, she began an ominous entry in her journal. "I'm not sure, but this may be the last time I write to you. I swallowed 15 (I think) Advils." A week earlier, she wrote, she had taken ten Advils and nothing had happened. But this time she wasn't sure. "I wish I could call one of my friends right now and say, 'I just took 15 Advils. Help me.'" But, she wrote, "I can't open up to anyone for fear that they'll betray me. That they wouldn't give two shits."

She followed that entry with a suicide note. It was addressed to "mom, dad, family, whoever the fuck reads this." She wrote: "I hate you. I especially hate *you,* mom and dad." We had ignored her pleas for help, and broken a promise to find her a therapist. Alicia was right about that. We had found out about her first suicide attempt when Liz picked up Alicia's journal one day and read a portion of it without asking her. We told Alicia we would find her a therapist. But when she seemed better, we let it drop. We hadn't learned much.

She went on to say good-bye to her friends, mentioning some of them by name. "You helped me in ways no one else could," she wrote to one. "You're the only person I could confide in about my first suicide attempt," she told another. "The rest of my Ridgewood friends, we had fun, didn't we?" She saved her final good-byes for her family. "Mom and dad, I did love you sometimes," she wrote. "Alex and Matt, you were great in my life. I love you two very much." She said good-bye to our Scottish Terrier, Reggie, and ended with "Goodnight and goodbye." She wrote her name, and drew a heart around it. Then she added, "P.S. Dad, take care of mom."

In such circumstances the same question always arises: Was it a serious suicide attempt or a cry for help? If it was a cry for help, it wasn't a very effective one. Alicia didn't leave a suicide note where we could immediately find it. She wrote it in her journal, where we wouldn't have looked unless her suicide attempt had been successful. If this had been a cry for help, I reasoned, she would have let us know what was happening, so that we could rescue her, and so that we would get the message that she was in grave trouble. But she didn't let us know, so I was forced to conclude that it was a serious suicide attempt. The next entry in her journal was nearly a month later: "So here I am, alive," she wrote. "I woke the next morning with a massive headache as a reminder, but I was alive. God, isn't the word *alive* great. The feeling of being ALIVE. Thank you, thank you god. I know someone was watching over me because here I am."

The night before, Alicia had slept over at a close friend's house, and she had told her friend about the Advils. She told her friend about the cutting, too, and showed her the angry crosshatch of scars on her upper arms and also on her belly. Alicia's friend urged her to tell her counselor at school. "But I don't think I want to," Alicia wrote. "I don't want to endure my parents and therapy."

In December, once again, I received a call at the office. This time it came from the principal at Alicia's middle school. Alicia was with her counselor in the guidance office. The principal and her counselor believed she was in immediate danger of harming herself. They had already called the police to pick her up. I didn't understand. Yes, she had been out of sorts, but I couldn't believe she would hurt herself. At the time, I knew nothing about the suicide attempt in November. I didn't think it possible that Alicia could be capable of suicide, or could even think about it. She was only twelve years old. How could she acquire enough grief and despair in only twelve years to consider killing herself?

Alicia's friend had told her parents about the Tylenol, the Advil, and the cutting. After considering this revelation for a while, they had decided to call the principal. I wish they'd called us, but I suppose they felt they couldn't face us, or maybe they thought we wouldn't take it seriously. Maybe that call was just too hard to make: "Hi, how are you? I'm just calling because I thought you should know that your daughter recently tried to commit suicide, and she's cutting herself . . ."

It was a devastating blow. I felt responsible, again, as I had so often with Alex. How could I have missed the scars left by the razor blade? I'd seen Alicia get into and out of her pajamas. She hadn't made any obvious attempt to cover herself up in the summer. Again, one of my children was in an emotional crisis, and, again, I'd missed it.

The police met Alicia at school, and Liz took her home. When I got the call at work, I was in the final day of editing a series of stories, a job that couldn't be handed off to another editor at that late stage. I wanted to grab my coat, run to the elevator, and catch the earliest train. But I couldn't. I had to finish the work. My own editor was away and couldn't take over for me. Nobody else on the staff had any expertise in the subject that the stories covered. I was stuck there. It felt wrong. But I didn't know what else to do. I single-mindedly focused on the stories, and finished several hours later. Then I ran for the train.

When I got home later that night, Liz and Alicia had been there for several hours. The house was dark and tense. That afternoon, Liz had called Psychiatrist No. 6, who was no longer treating Alex, and asked whether he could see Alicia right away. He agreed to meet with her the next day.

When Alicia went to see him, she told him about the suicide attempts and the cutting. She had been cutting herself almost every night at the beginning of the school year, but she had stopped in October, she told him, because she didn't want anyone to find out.

That same evening, Alicia took a shower after dinner. She had been standing under the water for only a few minutes when she began screaming frantically for her mother. "I'm afraid I'm going to cut myself," she said, sobbing. Liz helped her out of the shower and helped her dry herself and put on her pajamas. We watched her carefully until she fell asleep. We slept off and on, checking on her frequently during the night. Alex seemed to be deeply affected. He was concerned, and perhaps also a little relieved that, for once, he was not at the center of a family crisis. He made it a project to collect all the razors, scissors, and medicines in the house that Alicia might use to hurt herself. Liz put them in a couple of plastic bags and hid them.

The next day, we called Psychiatrist No. 6 again and told him what had happened. He concluded that Alicia should be hospitalized immediately. He began calling to see whether he could find a place for her.

This was always a tense time, waiting, with a child in a critical situation, to see whether a hospital bed would be available. I didn't understand why this seemed to happen every time one of the kids needed to be in the hospital. Once again, I felt it was important that I use my professional contacts to try to learn why finding a hospital bed was such an ordeal.

I made a few calls and did a little reporting, and I discovered that this was a problem not just in Ridgewood, or in the New York area, but all over the country. The U.S. psychiatric hospital system is on the verge of collapse, largely as a result of pressure from insurance companies and the federal government's Medicare and Medicaid programs. All over the country, psychiatric hospitals and psychiatric wards are going out of business. The beds are emptied, the white-coated doctors and nurses leave, the windows are shuttered and the doors locked. The fortunate patients return to their families, who have no alternative but to do the best they can to take care of their sick kin. Imagine the outcry if breast cancer patients were thrown out of the hospital, or victims of heart attacks or strokes. This is happening to psychiatric patients every day, yet we hear nothing about it on the news, in the papers, in the statehouses, or in the chambers of the U.S. Congress. Not one word.

Mark Covall, the executive director of the National Association of Psychiatric Health Systems, which represents psychiatric hospitals, gave me some of the statistics. Occupancy rates for children and adolescents in psychiatric hospitals and general hospitals with mental health units rose by just over 30 percent in the five-year period from 1997 to 2001, to the highest levels ever. In 2001, the occupancy rate for children's beds reached 65.4 percent. For adolescents, the figure was 68.9 percent. That's the average rate, but it fluctuates from day to day. Frequently, the hospitals will be full, and psychiatrists will not be able to find a place even for children who are in dire need of emergency care. Children's units are often small, with perhaps ten or twenty beds, so the difference between 65 percent occupancy and 100 percent occupancy may be only a few beds. The situation is worse in residential treatment centers, where children are often sent when they are discharged from psychiatric facilities. The residential treatment centers are intended as a bridge between hospitalization and a return home. Their occupancy rates ranged from 80 percent to 90 percent in 2001. Part of the reason for these high occupancy rates is that private psychiatric hospitals have been quickly going out of business. There were 460 such hospitals across the United States in 1995, but that number fell in 2002 by 42 percent, to only 265 private psychiatric hospitals serving the fifty states.

The exact causes of the decline are not clear, but it is clear that the hospitals could not make enough money to continue operating. One likely reason was a steep reduction in reimbursements by commercial insurance companies. A decade earlier, Covall said, 6 percent of all health care reimbursements went to mental health care. That proportion had fallen to 3 percent. In 1988, children and adolescents stayed in psychiatric hospitals for an average of more than forty days. By 2001, the average had fallen to about ten days. Those figures would be encouraging if they reflected an improvement in the treatment of mental illness, but they don't. They reflect a tightening in the amount of money available for mental health care, Covall said. Managed care's spending restrictions have hit care for mental health far harder than other medical care. "A lot of money has left the behavioral health care system," Covall told me. "There was more and more pressure to reduce costs, and hospitals did that. Psychiatric hospitals closed or merged with general hospitals. In the late 1990s, the general hospital behavioral health care units were closing as well. The number of beds has definitely declined. For kids, the problem is acute. General hospitals have not focused on kids, and with the freestanding psychiatric hospitals closing, there is a real crisis. The only option many people have is to go to an emergency room. And many emergency rooms are not staffed for a psychiatric emergency." The typical hospital emergency room does not have doors that will lock (to prevent a psychotic child from escaping) or guards to watch over potentially violent young patients.

The situation in public mental health systems is at least as bad. According to Dr. Paul S. Appelbaum, chair of the psychiatry department at the University of Massachusetts

Medical School and director of the university's law and psychiatry program, the states, in 2002, spent 30 percent less on mental health care, adjusted for inflation, than they had in 1955. Appelbaum, who was president of the American Psychiatric Association in 2002, noted that more state hospitals closed in the five years from 1990 to 1995 than in the twenty years before that. "The moral obligation of a just society to provide for the needs of the less fortunate . . . teeters on a precipice," Appelbaum told the annual meeting of the American Psychiatric Association in 2002. "Wishing that mental illness would not exist has led our policy makers to shape a health care system as if it did not exist."

I called the American Academy of Child and Adolescent Psychiatry, and I discovered that the problem of too few psychiatric hospitals is aggravated by a severe shortage of child psychiatrists. In 1990, a committee of medical school educators reviewed the data on mental illness in children and concluded that the nation would need 30,000 child psychiatrists by the year 2000. There are now about 6,300 child psychiatrists in the United States, and the number hasn't changed in a decade. Residency programs have the capacity to train nearly 900 new child psychiatrists every year, but during the past few years, only about 700 of those 900 slots for psychiatry residents have been filled. In some areas of the country, the shortage of child psychiatrists is particularly acute. Massachusetts has the largest number of child psychiatrists of any state—one for every 5,300 children. But children in rural and poor communities have far less access to psychiatric care. In Mississippi, the state at the bottom of the list, there is one child psychiatrist for every 125,000 children. New Jersey is somewhere in the middle.

The shortage of child psychiatrists may reflect, in part, the steep decline of American psychiatry during the past half century. In the years of relative peace and prosperity after World War II, American psychiatry was in the grip of Freud and psychoanalysis, and it offered the promise of a new science of mind. That was an exciting era. The brightest medical school graduates competed fiercely for psychiatric residencies. At the same time, however, researchers were laying the groundwork for a revolutionary change that would send psychiatry into a tailspin. A new generation of psychiatric drugs appeared. Among them were Thorazine, Valium, and Mellaril, the drug Alex was given. For the first time, psychiatrists could complement psychoanalysis and other forms of therapy with medications that had a profound effect on mental illness. Not all patients responded, and the medicines had serious side effects, but many psychiatric patients found that the drugs cleared their heads and allowed them to begin to take control of their lives. As the drugs proved their effectiveness, they began to supplant talk therapy, psychoanalysis, counseling, and behavioral treatments. Psychiatrists were losing the opportunity to engage with patients as they increasingly turned to writing prescriptions. Psychiatry steadily shed its allure. Now, most applicants for psychiatric residencies are in the bottom quarter of their medical school graduating classes. Most residencies are filled by foreign medical school graduates, which seems undesirable in a profession that still relies heavily on talking as a way to diagnose and treat illness. Foreign medical school graduates who come from another culture and may not be fluent in English may be very capable doctors, but they are unlikely to make good therapists.

Another reason for the precipitate decline of psychiatry

may be the wrenching changes forced upon it by managed care. Increasingly, therapy is done by social workers and psychologists, whose hourly rate is about half that of psychiatrists. The job that remains for psychiatrists is writing prescriptions. Managed care gives them as little as twenty minutes to assess a patient, decide on a treatment, and write the prescription. The message is, if you want to do serious therapeutic work with children, study clinical psychology or social work, not psychiatry. And that message is getting through: While residencies in psychiatry go unfilled, training programs in clinical psychology have twenty applicants for each position.

It's conceivable that pediatricians and family practitioners could fill some of the gap. American children make 150 million visits to pediatricians each year; that is often their only contact with the health care system. Parents trust their children's pediatricians and are likely to take their advice. Children with mental health problems are far more likely to see a pediatrician than a social worker, psychologist, or psychiatrist. But few pediatricians have any substantial training in child psychiatry. One third of American medical students have only minimal exposure to child psychiatry during medical school, internship, and residency.

The lack of training is not the only issue. Even if pediatricians knew what to look for, they don't have time to find it: The average pediatric visit lasts eleven to fifteen minutes. Even so, a significant number of children getting treatment are getting it from pediatricians and family practitioners. Most prescriptions for psychiatric drugs for children and adolescents are written by pediatricians, despite their lack of training.

Combine the drastic shortage of child psychiatrists with

the nearly total inability of pediatricians to help mentally ill kids, and who is left to provide care for these children? In millions of cases, the answer is: nobody.

A few hours after we'd talked to Psychiatrist No. 6, he called back to say that he had found a bed for Alicia at Four Winds, the hospital where Alex had been in the spring. We packed a bag of Alicia's clothes and drove her there. She was nervous and withdrawn. But she seemed to understand that she needed to be in the hospital; she didn't protest. We sat in the admissions office and signed a dozen consent forms, and then we sat through an interview with the admitting psychiatrist. Alicia told Liz and me, for the first time, about the suicide attempt. She talked about the cutting, and about the emotions that had an unyielding grip on her, the despair, and the terror of facing another day at school. The hospital's diagnosis was "depressive disorder NOS" (not otherwise specified). That is, her illness did not fit into any of the several recognized subcategories of depression. It was depression; no qualifiers needed.

We walked with Alicia to her unit, in the same building that Alex had been in. We kissed her, said good-bye, and heard the door close. I should have felt anger, sorrow, empathy—something. But I was drained. Again, I had heard that lock turn, and now it was my daughter who was apart from me. And I missed her. That was all I felt; I wanted her home. My feelings about putting the kids in the hospital had begun to change. I knew now that the worst time was the time just before the hospitalization. Alicia would get better in the hospital, and until she did she would be safe, or safer than we could keep her at home. Suicides do occur in psychiatric hospitals, but I refused to think about that. Things would get better. She would be okay.

That night, I sat at the piano and played "Bring Him Home," from *Les Misérables*. Alicia and I would often sit at the piano, where I would play and we would both sing. The songs from *Les Miz* were favorites of ours. I had trouble keeping my eyes focused on the music and the words. I was only part of the way through the song when I broke down.

Whatever was happening with Alicia was different from what had afflicted Alex. What she was going through was, in some sense, a wildly magnified and distorted version of the emotional turmoil that all children undergo in middle school. Girls are especially susceptible to losing their emotional gyroscopes during these difficult years. Some stop eating, finding that the pain and hunger of anorexia draw energy away from their out-of-control emotions. Others engage in what is sometimes called the new anorexia or the alternative anorexia—a different way of using pain to deal with emotional turmoil: They cut themselves. How this provides comfort is something that I do not ever expect to understand. Sometimes cutting is accompanied by suicide, but often it is not. Self-mutilation is not failed suicide; it is something else.

I learned this from a book I'd stumbled across in a bookstore's psychology section, looking for something that might help me understand what was happening with Alicia. I didn't expect to find an entire book about people who deliberately hurt themselves, but there it was. It was called *Cutting*. I found the title repellent. When I opened it and began to read the stories of people, mostly adolescent girls, who were "self-mutilators," I was repelled by that term, too. The author,

Steven Levenkron, a therapist in New York City, begins the book with stories of girls who cut themselves, story after story of behavior that seems incomprehensible to those of us who shiver at the thought of a paper cut, to say nothing of a razor blade slicing into soft flesh. I almost put the book down; it was difficult to continue reading. Levenkron begins the book that way deliberately, to make a point: "The self-mutilator is looked upon with fear, anger, disgust and revulsion." Therapists often feel that way, too, he writes, when their patients engage in this behavior. The point of Levenkron's graphic stories is to make cutting more familiar, to try to ease the disgust and revulsion that it inspires. "Desensitizing ourselves to the behaviors and the scars they inflict does not mean desensitizing ourselves to the patient's emotional distress. It is, rather, the first step necessary to seeing the self-mutilator for what she is: a person in desperate need of help and human contact."

I didn't need to be desensitized to know that Alicia was in desperate need of help. I never regarded her with disgust or revulsion, or anger. I was afraid for her, and I didn't understand the link between cutting and suicide, if there was one. Levenkron said they were different, and other researchers agreed. But Alicia was suicidal, too. The two things together were almost too much to bear. Alex was finally doing better. I thought we were going to get back on track. And now we had discovered that Alicia had been suffering, alone, for months. When she admitted to the psychiatrist that she'd been cutting herself, she wasn't shy about showing us the scars we'd missed during those long months. Her shoulders were crisscrossed with short, jagged, irregular marks, like the scribblings of an infant with a crayon. It was heartbreaking to look at them.

The day that Alicia was admitted to the hospital, we met

with her therapist there. She talked about her feelings of depression, and about her suicide attempts. She said she didn't want to hurt herself, but that she was afraid she might do so again. During the next two days, she told her therapist that she still had a desire to hurt herself, but that she had not acted on it. On her third day in the hospital, the therapist was already making plans for her release.

Alicia took her journal along with her, and her observations reflect her resignation to the situation. "So, lots has happened since I wrote to you. I'm sitting on my bed in a mental hospital. Surprisingly, it's not that bad . . ."

Alicia got along well with the other patients in the hospital, but still reported having suicidal thoughts. She was put on the fifteen-minute watch list; someone from the staff had to check at least every fifteen minutes to be sure she was safe, and make a notation to that effect in Alicia's chart. The next day, she became argumentative and refused to comply with the staff's requests. But by the evening, she was calm again. In her group sessions, she became more willing to talk about her cutting and about the feelings of worthlessness that went along with it. She said she regretted cutting and didn't plan to do it anymore. And that was the way her hospital stay continued. She would have occasional thoughts of hurting herself, and she would appear withdrawn during some of the group activities, and then she would brighten and improve.

We visited Alicia every day, just as we had Alex. We would bring the usual Chinese food or pizza, or sometimes a bucket of chicken. We would stop first at the nurses' station, where our bags had to be checked for any dangerous or contraband items. It wasn't firearms or explosives they were looking for, but mundane items that the patients might use to hurt themselves or threaten one another. The Cokes had to be in paper cups; cans and bottles were not allowed on the unit. Actually, Cokes weren't allowed, either. Only noncaffeinated beverages: caffeine-free sodas, or fruit juice. No gum. We were not allowed to bring food for any of the other patients with whom Alicia had made friends. Socializing with them was strongly discouraged, beyond a quick hello. Cameras were not allowed, to protect patient privacy. And no cigarettes. (When Alex was admitted to Four Winds, cigarettes were used as rewards for good behavior. Patients who followed the rules during the morning were allowed to step out at midday for a cigarette break. That struck me as a bizarre policy, using addiction to a dangerous drug to help kids recover from mental illness. By the time we had returned with Alicia, smoking had been banned in the hospital.) I understood the reasons for these rules, and the staff was gracious in enforcing them. But I always felt a little uneasy: How could they think that Liz or I would bring Alicia items that might be harmful? Admittedly, I wouldn't have thought to eliminate some of the banned items; I wasn't accustomed to thinking of a soda can as a deadly weapon.

Exactly one week after her admission, Alicia was discharged. One of the nurses pronounced her "in good health," and wrote, in the parlance of medicine, that Alicia "denies wanting to hurt herself." She was, however, "anxious about discharge," the nurse added. Alicia told her therapist that if she had further thoughts about hurting herself, she would not act on them. She promised to tell her parents or her school counselor if she had such thoughts. The therapist concluded his report by saying that the "patient presented no imminent risk for suicidal or homicidal behavior."

Alicia had mixed feelings about leaving. "I'm happy and upset at the same time," she wrote in her journal. "I mean, no one wants to be in a mental institution, but I feel so safe and secure here. There are no pressures, and everybody loves and understands one another. We all look past skin color and hairdos to the person buried inside, screaming for help."

Alicia seemed much better the evening we took her home. She had been given the antidepressant Paxil in the hospital, but that couldn't have kicked in yet. A week wasn't enough time. She was happy again, no longer overwhelmed by the thoughts of self-harm and suicide that had frightened her so badly and had led to her hospitalization. But how could she have been better? What could have happened in one week to quell emotional troubles that had been building up for months or longer? Alex had seemed improved each time he left the hospital, too, but that didn't always last.

We began to look for a therapist for Alicia after her discharge, but we weren't fast enough. In early January 2000, less than a month after she left the hospital, Alicia talked to one of the friends she'd made there. "We talked about how we'd cut ourselves since we got home (yes, I have)," she wrote in her diary. And she continued: "I really hate my parents right now. I'm not sure why, but that's why I cut myself. I HATE them. I need someone to talk to. Someone who won't send me back to the hospital. That's why I don't want a therapist. They'll make me go back."

In February 2000, when she was in the seventh grade, Alicia began seeing a social worker in Ridgewood. One of the things the therapist wanted was to determine why Alicia was cutting herself. So far, Alicia had been diagnosed as depressed and had been treated for depression. But was her illness really depression, or something else? Even though her symptoms and circumstances were different from Alex's, could she have some variant of bipolar disorder? The attack by the other girls at school clearly played a role in her illness, but would it alone have driven her to attempt suicide? Besides, that was over now, and Alicia hadn't recovered. Something else was going on.

I was confused, too, and disappointed in myself. I was trying hard to be more understanding. I'd started to read and to learn more about Alex's illness. I'd talked to psychiatrists, psychologists, and others, in my role as a reporter, trying to learn whatever I could. And I was reexamining everything I thought I knew about being a father. I was trying hard to understand what was happening with Alicia, but her situation was different enough from Alex's that I wasn't sure anything I'd learned so far was relevant to her.

The new therapist noted that Alicia was doing better in school, but that she had problems controlling her temper. She was "oppositional" with her parents and had "some identity confusion," as well as increased impulsivity and anxiety. She "is struggling to achieve some degree of independence, which appears appropriate but difficult for parents to accept." In one session that I attended with Alicia, we talked about how much we enjoyed each other's company, and we joked about what a good relationship we had. I was happy to sit in the therapist's office and talk about that, because I felt good about it. With all the trouble Alicia was having, we had at least kept that together: we could still talk, and we could agree to disagree about whether she was spending enough time on homework or too much time with her friends. I was proud of Alicia for the way she could express herself, and for the maturity she showed in these sessions, and I was proud of our relationship. The boys' entry into adolescence had meant that they needed to separate themselves from me, try out their legs, test their independence. Alicia didn't seem to need that. She seemed able to taste a little independence without needing to push me away.

After seeing Alicia almost weekly for several months, the therapist concluded that Alicia was suffering not from depression, but from borderline personality disorder. Which is what? I asked her. I'd never heard of it. It sounded like something not quite real, not a genuine disorder, but a "borderline" one, on the line between normal and abnormal. That was how I heard it.

The therapist did her best to explain, but still I didn't understand. I went back to the bookstore to look for help. By now, I had acquired a shelf full of books pertaining to Alex's and Alicia's current and former diagnoses. Every time a new diagnosis came up, I'd pick up two or three books. I'd get partway through them before being told that that diagnosis was wrong; some therapist or psychiatrist had come up with a new one. And I'd run out and buy two or three more books. I was having trouble keeping up.

One hallmark of borderline personality disorder is self-mutilation. Some people with the illness cut or burn themselves. That was what had led the therapist to suspect this diagnosis in Alicia. But borderline personality disorder is more than that. Its characteristics include unstable personal relationships and moods and impulsive behavior. Its victims suffer from excessive fear of abandonment, feelings of emptiness, sudden anger, and periodic episodes of depression or anxiety that can last for hours or days. They can be extremely needy, and yet can turn quickly on anyone who responds to that need. Their impulsive behaviors include such things as binge eating, drinking, drug abuse, spending and shoplifting. And they are frequently suicidal.

Some of this sounded right. Alicia was suicidal; she was cutting herself. I didn't see the anxiety, emptiness, and fear of abandonment, but I wasn't going to second-guess the therapist. Maybe this was it. And maybe now that we had a diagnosis, we could find appropriate treatment for Alicia.

A few months later, Alicia decided she'd had enough of that therapist, and she stopped going. She refused to see anyone else. Nobody ever mentioned borderline personality disorder again. The diagnosis had gone nowhere. I put a few more unfinished books on my shelf.

In early June, Alicia, now thirteen, called Liz from school one day, saying she felt weak and dizzy and couldn't stand up. She was nauseated, her head ached terribly, and she felt extremely tired. Liz took her to the pediatrician, who said Alicia should go to the emergency room. There, because of her past hospitalization and suicide attempts, she was given a careful look. A neurologist was brought in to examine her. Neither the neurologist nor the emergency room doctors could find anything wrong. Alicia was soon sitting up, eating crackers and peanut butter, and telling them she felt much better. She was discharged with instructions to rest, and to return if the symptoms reappeared.

Before she left, however, she told a social worker that she was still cutting herself on the arms and stomach with a razor blade. In routine questioning, she denied using drugs, but admitted that she drank "occasionally." The last time she'd had alcohol was the previous weekend. The social worker didn't say anything about Alicia's alcohol use, perhaps because she felt that would be a violation of Alicia's right to confidentiality, and because it would likely mean the end of the therapy. It would have been nice to know that Alicia, at the age of thirteen, was "experimenting" with alcohol, or was perhaps already beyond experimentation. A little parental intervention there would have been a good thing. It's not entirely clear whether the social worker was correct to withhold the information. Some therapists have told me that I have a right to know what's going on with my children, at least until they are eighteen. But rarely did they volunteer about alcohol or drug use on the part of either Alex or Alicia. It's a sensitive issue, not only because of the harm that drugs and alcohol can do to kids, or the legal difficulties that can arise, but also because these drugs can interfere with the proper working of psychiatric medications. In some cases, it was difficult to get copies of Alicia's and Alex's psychiatric records while I was working on this book, even when the kids had signed releases allowing me to see them. It's hard to know what is right. Confidentiality is important, too, so that the kids will be willing to open up to their therapists.

With the end of the school year, Alicia improved. She spent four weeks at a YMCA summer camp where she'd gone before. The counselors made sure she took her antidepressant medications, and Alicia returned home happy and, apparently, healthy. A few years earlier, I would have been eager to latch on to that. I would have swept away my concerns, and decided that the troubling episode was over. I knew better than that now. I had learned, after deceiving myself for years about Alex, that these things couldn't be willed or wished away. I hoped Alicia was better. I hoped she'd gone through the worst of it, and that she would settle in to school in the fall and feel good about it and about herself. But I knew that was not a sure thing.

Alicia began eighth grade with enthusiasm. She'd always liked school, enjoyed being with her friends, looked forward to her new classes each fall, and been an excellent student when she wasn't struggling under the burden of her emotional difficulties. That burden had been eased, but not yet lifted. It was still unclear what was happening with Alicia emotionally, and there was no reason to think that anyone had reached to the core of her troubles. She had stopped seeing the therapist around the end of the previous school year. She saw Psychiatrist No. 6 only occasionally, not enough for him to take her emotional temperature or engage her in therapy. Like Alex, she had been expelled from the health care system, without a diagnosis and without any idea where she was headed. Was she at risk of another emotional slide? Would she be likely to start cutting herself again, or was that safely behind us? Should we continue to surreptitiously scan her shoulders for fresh scars?

The mental health system had given us no answers to those questions, but it became apparent, soon enough, that not much had changed. Once Alicia was back in school, she began to decline. Her grades dropped, as did her motivation, her energy, and her view of herself. I couldn't tell whether she was heading toward another crisis, but she certainly wasn't getting better. Neither Liz nor I knew what to do to head off what might be coming, so we didn't do much of anything. We watched.

Within a few weeks, Alicia was in danger of failing her courses. Her counselor met with her to discuss the situation.

Alicia used the occasion not to discuss school, but as an opportunity for an emotional outpouring. She quickly began to talk about cutting. She told the counselor she had been cutting herself for three years, far longer than any of us had suspected. Mostly she would use a knife or razor to try to get some "relief" when she was angry or upset. Some days, however, she would cut herself when she was feeling good. She thought the cutting might intensify the good feelings. She said she had been depressed for about four years, and that she had lost interest in school around the middle of the seventh grade. She had played soccer and a year of lacrosse, but she said she lost interest in sports, too, around the same time she lost interest in school. I wondered whether all of this could be right. Had she really been cutting herself for three years? Or was she misremembering? I didn't understand how it could have gone on that long without Liz or me noticing the scars. But teenagers are very private about their bodies. Whether she had been cutting herself for one year or three, she had evidently been clever enough to conceal it from us.

Alicia's counselor put her through a series of tests to assess her academic ability. She was cooperative but passive, offering few comments beyond what the testing required. She seemed sad and resigned, he thought. In a variety of tests of her cognitive skills, her scores ranged from average to above average. In a test in which she was asked to remember and repeat a string of digits forward and backward, "Alicia accomplished something I had never seen in many years," her counselor wrote. "That is, she was able to recall eight digits and present them in reverse order on two trials. This revealed a tremendous capacity for powerful concentration, mental manipulation of information, and short-term auditory memory."

I was surprised to learn that Alicia did less well on another test, one intended to assess verbal expression, knowledge of social conventions, and judgment. She was articulate and perceptive enough to understand social norms for someone her age, I would have thought. Her counselor attributed her poor performance to "a somewhat passive attitude to responding to questions . . . as well as a lack of awareness of effective social behavior." An emotional assessment confirmed that Alicia was, indeed, clinically depressed, but the test's results were not uniformly bleak. The assessment also showed that she was interested in having fun with her friends. Unlike some people who are depressed, she had not lost all interest in pleasant activities.

On Columbus Day weekend, Alicia asked for permission to go away for a few days with a friend, Allison. We knew Allison well, and we knew her parents, who were divorced but who both lived nearby. We consented. The trip would be a good way for her to escape the pressure at school. Maybe she would be able to regroup and recapture a little of the enthusiasm with which she'd begun the school year. Allison's brother, who was Alex's age, brought a friend, too, a popular kid named Brian, who was also a friend of Alex's. I'd met him briefly only a week or two before. He was friendly and polite, and seemed like a nice kid. The kids took off to Allison's father's weekend house, a few hours' drive from Ridgewood, near the beach. We didn't hear from Alicia while she was away, but when she came back, lugging a backpack full of damp, sandy clothes, she said she'd had a good time. It had been fun. There wasn't much point in probing further. If she wanted to tell us more, she would. If not, no amount of persuasion would get it out of her.

Two days later, I was at home about ten in the evening, getting ready for bed upstairs, when I heard some commotion downstairs in the living room. I went down to find the mother of one of Alicia's friends standing there. She was agitated. I tried to take in the scene. I hardly knew this woman. What was she doing walking into my house? "What's going on?" I asked. Alicia walked in behind the woman, with her head hung down. She folded herself into an easy chair, fidgeting and looking down at her hands.

"Alicia's been raped," the woman said. "I've called the police. They'll be here in a few minutes."

I took a step back. This person had called the police before discussing the situation with me or with Liz. I was too stunned to be outraged. Before I could begin to register what she'd said, a policeman stepped in the front door.

"Are you Mr. Raeburn?" he asked.

"Yes," I said. "Can you tell me what's happening?"

"We got a call that your daughter had been the victim of a sexual assault," he said. He looked down at Alicia, and back to me. "Is this your daughter?"

A few minutes later, we were all at the Ridgewood police station. Allison's mother showed up with her boyfriend. So did Allison's father and his wife. Liz and I were both there. And so was the woman who had called the police; she had, inexplicably, followed us to the station. I couldn't understand why she was there. It seemed she had done us a favor, although Alicia hadn't given Liz or me any indication that there had been trouble over the weekend. Now Alicia had apparently confided in this woman, a stranger to me. I was hurt, but I was trying to tell myself not to worry about that; at least we had found out what happened. But why was this woman still here? Why had she called the police before calling us, so that we could make the decisions about what had to be done? Finally, I asked her to leave.

The rest of us sat for two hours in a closed room, around an ancient wooden table. The time crawled. The desk officer on duty had called a detective to come in and interview the girls, the beginning of the process of determining whether charges would be filed against the assailant. It was Brian, they said. The attack had happened during their weekend at the beach with Allison's father.

As we sat there, waiting, Allison and Alicia were strangely amused by all of this, giggling, drawing pictures on napkins, passing notes, and whispering. From time to time, one or the other of them would begin to cry softly, and the other would comfort her. They would hug. Sometimes, they stepped out of the room to talk.

The tension in the room was unbearable. We were angry, confused, and frightened. Allison's parents were at odds with each other over how this could have happened at Allison's father's house. The unspoken question was, Where were he and his wife when this took place?

We began, haltingly, to ask the girls what had happened, trying not to let our anger settle on them. The last night they were away, the four kids—Allison, Alicia, Allison's brother, and Brian—had gone to the beach for a little party. Brian brought a container of vodka. Allison's brother, uncomfortable because Brian seemed more interested in the girls than in him, turned back to the house and left Brian alone with the girls. Brian, who was seventeen at the time, brought out the vodka and made sure the girls, who were then fourteen, had plenty to drink. And then he sexually assaulted both of them on the beach, first one, then the other. They were too drunk to stop him, they said. But not too drunk to remember the pain, and the overwhelming sense of powerlessness, knowing what was happening but being unable to prevent it.

Each of them confessed to a deep sense of shame at being unable to protect the other. They had suffered not only the violation of the assault, but also the tragedy of watching it happen to a best friend.

At last the detective arrived. He finished interviewing the girls just before four A.M. We then took the girls to the local hospital's emergency room, where they could be examined. An hour later, a counselor from the local rape-crisis center showed up. She talked with the girls, both of whom seemed to find her helpful. We left the hospital at eight A.M.

Alicia told only a few very close friends about the assault. Maybe she thought it would remain a secret, or maybe not. But within a day or two the news was all over the school. For a time, the students seemed to sympathize with Allison and Alicia. But that changed, and soon many were defending Brian. This development played nicely into the hands of the girls who, in the sixth grade, had accused Alicia of being involved with most of the boys in the class. If they thought she was a "slut" then, well, now they had the proof. What was worse, Alicia now accepted the label. No taunting from the kids could have compared with the agonizing rebukes she was delivering to herself. "I'm sorry. I'm sorry I did this to everyone," she wrote in her journal. "People have their own problems without having me add to them. Sometimes I wish I hadn't told anyone. . . . All I know is that I'm trying my hardest to be strong."

It was several days before Alicia could face going back to school. She knew that word had spread, and she didn't know what kind of reception she would get. When she did go back, a boy she'd known since kindergarten blamed Alicia for the assault and expressed sympathy for Brian. "Why did you get him in trouble? If I were you, I'd be happy." Some friends were horrified. Others embellished the story as they passed it along, telling tales about Alicia and Allison confronting Brian in court. Brian was telling people that Alex's little sister had encouraged his advances, that it was her fault. "From what my brother tells me, most people are believing Brian," Alicia wrote in her journal. "Alex Raeburn's life was ruined by his little sister. She is sorry."

A few nights later, Alicia wrote in her journal, "I'm not a slut! I'm not a slut! I'm not a slut! Maybe if I say it enough, it'll come true." She reached for her razor. "Blood came. All the pain's going away. . . . Bye-bye Brian. . . . Have fun in hell. Cause that's where you've put me. I hope you enjoy it as much as I do."

Months later, Alicia was still agonizing, still blaming herself for the events of that evening: "I'm sitting here crying about what I've gone through. What about what I let happen to Allison? What about what I've put my family through? It's all my fault. I swear it. I'm going away. . . ."

A few days after the assault, Brian was charged with six counts of sexual misconduct and one count of sexual abuse. Alicia noted the lack of a rape charge. Didn't the police believe her, either?

Several years later, I found out that Brian had met a little vigilante justice. Three or four days after word of the rape spread through the high school, a group of students pounced on Brian after school and beat him badly enough that they were charged with assault. Some of the attackers were friends of Alex and of Allison's older brother, who felt they had to do what the two boys didn't dare because of the punishment they could face. The attack occurred on school grounds, so the disciplinarian at the high school got involved. He told the students who were responsible that he would do what he could to make it easy on them, because Brian had deserved what he got. Even so, several were charged, and one was put on probation. But none of this was ever discussed publicly. Brian left the high school a week later.

Ridgewood had a pattern of keeping such disturbing events under wraps. It wouldn't be good for property values if potential buyers heard about rapes of young girls or vigilante justice administered by high school students. A few years before, the town had taken a beating in the press when charges were filed against four Ridgewood high school students for gang-raping a high school freshman. The rape was covered up for two weeks, until the local press got wind of it. To make matters worse, two more Ridgewood high school students were charged with witness tampering after they threatened the victim with physical violence if she testified against her attackers.

The high school kids say it's not unusual for a teenager in Ridgewood to carry a knife. Some of them have guns. Marijuana, cocaine, and crack are easy to find, and heroin use is growing, the kids say. One boy who had a long history of trouble with his divorced parents lived on the streets in Ridgewood for months, sleeping in a basement room he broke into and eating what he found in Dumpsters. But none of this is ever discussed. When the school system issued a memorandum to parents on its implementation of President George Bush's No Child Left Behind Act, it said not a word about addressing problems of violence or drugs in the district. Instead, in a thrilling example of cluelessness, it proclaimed, "All children are viewed as 'Village Treasures' and will be provided the opportunity to reach their highest potential as learners."

The village itself, for its part, didn't do any better than the school system at recognizing the realities in Ridgewood. "Ridgewood is recognized as an exceptional residential community," says the chamber of commerce. "Villagers live in distinctive homes set back on quiet, tree-lined streets. Homes and public areas are maintained with a strong sense of personal and community pride." This brochure goes on to say that a national magazine recently described Ridgewood "as one of the safest towns in America." Maybe so for the town's Wall Street wizards, but less true, it seems, for their children.

It was difficult to know, at the time, how Alex was reacting to Alicia's increasingly serious emotional problems. He didn't say much, and I think he didn't mind having the focus off him for a while. He continued to fight with his brother, on occasion, and when Matt would become angry, Alex demanded to know why Matt wasn't required to undergo psychiatric care. Before Alicia got sick, Alex had a vague sense that he was being unfairly dealt with, that his brother and sister had emotional problems, too, but that they weren't "punished" with therapy, medication, and hospitalization.

But the rape had a huge effect on Alex. The assailant was a friend of his; Alex had once introduced us when we ran into Brian on the sidewalk in Ridgewood. Alex saw the rape as a profound betrayal by his friend. And the kids Alex's age immediately divided into two camps: those who saw Brian as unfairly accused by a girl who, more or less, had it coming; and those who were loyal to Alex, ready to go after Brian whenever and wherever they could. For years afterward, Alex worried that he would run into Brian at a party and that he might do something he would regret. And they did run into each other on a couple of occasions, but the situation was defused before anything happened. It was a brutally tense standoff, and a huge burden on Alex.

A month after the sexual assault, Alicia walked into a JCPenney store in a nearby mall, wandered through the girls' clothes awhile, and then walked out with a sweatshirt. She was spotted immediately. A store detective grabbed her, handcuffed her, and called the police. They called Liz at home. "I really screwed up this time," Alicia wrote in her diary. "I wonder if my parents will ever forgive me." She couldn't say why she had done it. "I don't know who I am anymore," she wrote. "But there is one thing I do know . . . she's not me."

A few days later, Alicia met with a juvenile officer at the county courthouse. Just when I was getting used to therapists, psychiatrists, and psychiatric hospitals, I now had the opportunity to try something new: accompanying one of my children on an encounter with the juvenile justice system. The court officer saw that she was not dealing with a child who was likely to become a career criminal, and so she dealt with Alicia rather gently. She pointed out that the consequences of any further shoplifting could be severe, and she extracted promises from Alicia that she would never do this again. She ordered Alicia to watch a videotape on the evils of shoplifting and to write a report on it. Alicia had a few weeks to do that. If she complied, the matter would be dropped, with nothing on her record.

I didn't know what to add to that. Liz decided that Alicia should be grounded "indefinitely," whatever that meant. For a few days, she kept Alicia on a very short leash, denying her use of the phone or her AOL e-mail account. And she told

Alicia that she would now have to undergo therapy again, making the therapy seem more like a threat than something that was supposed to be helpful. As it turned out, "indefinitely" didn't last more than a few days. Alicia was soon on her own again, meeting her friends in town or at their houses after school, when most parents were still at work.

And that wasn't the only notable event of the weeks immediately following the assault. Alicia had sex with her boyfriend for the first time. "You know what the crazy part is?" she wrote. "I'm not at all upset. I thought 13-year-olds that lost their virginity were supposed to be 'I wasn't ready.' But that's not the thing I'm feeling. I feel so excited and in love."

David had been Alicia's boyfriend since the seventh grade. I had often worried that he might be the cause of some of her distress. Tall, thin, and fair, he was a quiet boy, difficult to get to know. And he was rarely around the house. Alicia and he hung out together in town, in the park, or on a street corner, or they spent time at David's house. I wondered sometimes why they didn't spend more time at our house, but neither Alex nor Matt had spent much time with their friends there, either. As soon as they were old enough to be allowed to wander off our block, they rarely brought friends home. Was it because our house was smaller than most of the houses in Ridgewood? Perhaps the children felt cramped at our place, in our sight all the time. At their friends' houses, they could stretch out and relax in a downstairs rec room or an upstairs bedroom, watching movies and playing music without any family competition for the TV or the stereo. At our house, that was difficult. We had one TV, in the family room, and the kids' bedrooms were too small to hold more than one or two friends at a time. Whatever the reason, David was rarely around. (Later, both Alex and Alicia told me that one reason they stayed away was to avoid exposing their friends to the arguments between Liz and me.)

Although David went to a different school, everyone knew they were a couple. Did this reinforce the image of Alicia as sexually promiscuous? I didn't know whether she was sexually active with him, and I worried that, even at the age of thirteen, she might be. They were very affectionate, and she had no hesitation about giving him a kiss hello or good-bye in front of me, leaving me to wonder what else was happening when I wasn't watching. I suppose I could have asked her, but I didn't. I wasn't ready to face the answer. I told myself it was best not to cause problems and risk shutting off the good communication between us. I told myself that she wouldn't tell me the truth, anyway, so why should I ask? I was sure Alicia would come to me to talk about any problems she was having with David. I was understanding; I would be reasonable if she was reasonable.

There was the rub. There was no way that I was going to deem regular sexual activity at the age of thirteen reasonable, and I'm sure Alicia knew that. If she had told me the truth, what would I have done? I'd like to think I would have been understanding, would have explained why having sex so young wasn't a good idea, and would have expected her to understand and to stop. That's what I'd like to think, but I would be deceiving myself. I surely would not have calmly tried to explain the risks of early sexual activity. More likely, I would have told her I was outraged. And I would have told her she couldn't see David again. Furthermore, even if I had managed to remain calm—which, as Alicia knew, was unlikely—I doubt I could have persuaded her to stop. That was a *Leave It to Beaver* fantasy, me at my desk, like Ward

Cleaver, explaining to Alicia what she had done wrong, and warmly commending her for admitting she was wrong. "Gee, Dad, I'm sorry!" That wasn't very believable in the 1950s, and it certainly wasn't now.

If I had told her she couldn't see David anymore, how could I possibly have enforced the ban? I wasn't home until late, and Liz was far less likely than I was to try to enforce anything like that. Nor could we talk about it; I knew before even raising the question that whatever I decided, Liz would disagree. Why bother trying to formulate a plan? We would never get together on this. We never got together on anything.

Alicia's journals reveal how difficult the relationship was for her. David was unpredictable. He would yank her one way and then another, sending her reeling like the last person on line in crack-the-whip. He would leave her wounded, then come back just before she was about to give up on him.

One night in April, when David and Alicia were in the seventh grade, David called to say that he had cut himself the previous Saturday night, because he had been mad at Alicia. "Now I feel horrible," Alicia wrote. "I cut myself three times on my stomach." Blaming herself for David's cutting, she had cut herself to try to expiate the guilt. Sympathy cuts.

A few days later, she was on the phone with David for what seemed like an hour or longer. At that time, we had only one line and no cell phones. Alex wanted to make a call, and I didn't want the phone tied up all night, in case someone was trying to reach us. Besides, it was a school night. I went up to her room and told her she had to be off the phone by ten. Alex came in several times and yelled at her to get off the phone. I went up again at ten-thirty and told Alicia she had to hang up immediately. It was time for bed. No more excuses. "You don't make the rules, do you hear me? Get off the phone!"

"I wanted to tell him that the reason I didn't get off was because I fucking wanted to die," Alicia wrote in her journal later that night. "My mom then comes in and starts yelling at me about my window being open. . . . Then my dad comes in again and tells me I have to go to bed. . . . I think he really wants me to die because he seemed to come in and scream at me at the exact time I was feeling extremely suicidal. I hate him. I hate my family." David, she wrote, "was making me feel better, so I didn't get off the phone."

The preoccupation with suicide continued. A week later, it was David who was feeling suicidal. He called Alicia late at night and told her that she should take his money when he died, that he was going to jump off his balcony. Alicia ran downstairs to tell Matt. He woke up Liz, who got on the phone with David and tried to calm him. She told him he could come over to stay at our house if that helped. She asked to talk to his parents, but when David asked her not to, she didn't. The next morning, when I was told about all of this, I couldn't believe what she'd done. "What makes you think you know how to talk to a kid who's thinking of killing himself?" I said to her. "Why on earth didn't you tell his parents? What if he had killed himself? How would you feel if his parents blamed you for his death?" In the end, it was difficult to know how serious David was about the suicide threat. He'd told Liz that he couldn't come over to spend the night at our house because he was meeting one of his friends early the next morning to go skating.

In June, months before Alicia walked out of JCPenney

with the stolen sweatshirt, David and his friends had bragged to Alicia about their own shoplifting. They had gone to the local supermarket, David told her, and stolen a box of coins and bills intended to be donated to underprivileged children. "Now, I have no problem with stealing," Alicia wrote in her journal. "Hell, Saturday I stole practically the whole fucking mall." But she was outraged that David and his friends had stolen money intended for a worthy cause. "That's just wrong." Apparently, Alicia had taken things from stores before. She wasn't caught, and she never said a word about it.

Sometimes, Alicia and David had sex without a condom. On one of those occasions, Alicia told her mother. Liz grabbed Alicia and took her to the emergency room for the morning-after pill. "Me and my mom got into a fight," Alicia wrote. They were in the emergency room until one-thirty in the morning. Alicia was also given a pregnancy test. It took two hours for the results to come back. "Those were the longest two hours of my life," Alicia wrote later that night. "I was so petrified that the test would be positive. When it came back negative, I felt like crying." I was not at home when this happened, and neither Liz nor Alicia told me about it. I didn't find out until much later, when Alicia showed me the relevant passage in her diaries. Liz and I had fought often about whether I had as much right as she did to make decisions on behalf of the children. But she eventually changed her strategy. I couldn't fight her if she didn't tell me what was happening. Increasingly, therefore, she kept these things to herself. I was outraged, embittered—and powerless.

David was on the scene and off again, for another year. When Alicia called and his cell phone was off, she imagined he was with another girl. "How can I live if I don't get him back or if he's with another girl right now?" she wrote. "God, don't take away the one thing that gives my life meaning. Don't take David from me, please. I need him."

One night, she drifted off the subject of David to consider how her life might be different:

"I wonder what it's like to be an eighth grader that's not in love. That eats dinner with their family every night and comes home after school every day to do their homework. That tries to be good, and the only time they get in trouble is when their parents catch them on the phone after nine or when they eat a sweet before dinner. I wonder what it's like to wake up every morning with a smile on your face. What it's like to want to live and to do what your parents say? Tell me, what does it feel like to love yourself? How do you eat dinner and not go to the bathroom to throw it up? When you cry, why do you not have to see the sight of blood to calm you down? How do you live each day to the fullest and not cry yourself to sleep from regret of the day that has just passed? I wonder what it's like to not be me?"

Alicia hobbled along through the fall of eighth grade. Her performance in school was erratic. The physical and emotional trauma of the rape colored everything she did. A rape counselor visited Alicia several times, and she was in therapy briefly, but within a few months she refused to go. She continued to see the psychiatrist and take medication, but she never did get the counseling and psychological care she needed to recover from the assault. On occasion, when she needed to, she could summon her wits to do well on an exam or an essay. But mostly she did just enough to get by. Her moods swung up and down. School did not seem to be a source of unhappiness, yet she was unable to regain her equilibrium. She was distant and uncommunicative. It seemed clear that tumultuous things

were going on among her and her friends, but Alicia
wouldn't talk about any of it. I was afraid for her, but I
didn't know what to do.

I had reason to be afraid. The crisis came on December
28, near the end of Christmas vacation. Matt was back from
college. We'd been home during the holidays except for a
brief overnight visit to see some of Liz's relatives. I was in
New York that night. I got home around ten. As I walked
around the corner, coming from the train station, I saw the
blinking lights of a police car and ambulance on the street
near the house. I stepped more quickly. The front door of the
house was open. I saw the dark shapes of several police officers and emergency medical technicians standing on the
front porch. I ran inside.

Matt met me at the door and said Alicia was in trouble. I
walked around to the living room. Alicia was in an uphol-
stered chair in the living room, writhing, screaming nonsense words, and struggling to run. A couple of her friends,
a policeman, and Matt held her down in the chair. I guess
they were her friends; I'd never seen them before. "What the
hell is going on?" I yelled. "What is this?" One of the police
officers stepped between me and Alicia, and started to tell
me what was going on.

Alicia had been at David's house. The two of them were
upstairs, where he had given her a glass of vodka. When
she'd finished that and asked for more, he'd given her a glass
of whiskey. She became acutely intoxicated, and she cut her
left forearm and both wrists with a razor. David panicked
and called his parents, who were downstairs and unaware of
what was happening one flight up. David was standing on the
front porch, with a couple of other guys Alicia's age that I
didn't know. I went up to David, right up to him, a few inches
from his face. "What the hell were you thinking?" I asked

him. "You know she's depressed and she's been in the hospital. How could you give her all that alcohol to drink?"

Cowering, he said, "She asked me for it." I was boiling. He wasn't a bad kid, I didn't think. I didn't believe he would intentionally harm Alicia. But how could I possibly know? I didn't really know anything about him. David didn't talk much. He was polite, but much too withdrawn for me to be able to say I knew him, even a little.

I left David and the others and went back inside. Alicia was still writhing on the chair, still being held down by a couple of kids I didn't know. "Who are you people?" I shouted. "Who let you in here? Get out of my house!" I turned to the police. "Why aren't you doing something? Why did you let these kids in here? Let's get her to the emergency room!" They looked at me suspiciously, wondering whether they had another problem on their hands, not only the drunk teenager, but her father, too. And they were right to be concerned. I was close to becoming another problem. I'd walked home and found my house in chaos, my daughter out of her mind, and my wife trying to negotiate something with these strangers, trying to get them to help. "I don't want them to help. Get them out of here," I shouted. "We have to get Alicia to the hospital." I found David again. "I'll talk to you later," I told him.

Liz was trying to mediate somehow, talking to these kids, and talking to the police. As soon as I'd displayed my anger, she was yelling at me to stop it, telling me I was making things worse. It wasn't a message I was ready to accept. I wanted something done. Alicia should be the focus here. I remember several police officers standing around, and at least a couple of EMTs. Everybody seemed to be moving slowly, deliberately, far too slowly and deliberately for what was an obvious emergency. And who were these damn kids?

The kids finally started to wander away, in a group, after what seemed like nearly an hour, although it might have been less than half of that. The EMTs wheeled a gurney into the living room, strapped Alicia to it, bundled her into the ambulance, and drove off. Liz, Matt, and I got in the car and followed.

Alex wasn't home during this crisis. And that was fine with him. Increasingly, he had separated himself from the arguments between Liz and me, from his brother, and from Alicia, feeling that he needed to tend to his own problems and couldn't take on anything else. He continued to be deeply disturbed by the rape, but otherwise he did everything he could to distance himself from the family, where each crisis seemed to lead to another. He spent as much time as possible away from the house, at friends' houses or cruising around town in somebody's car. I thought then, and still think, that he was doing the right thing. After years of trying to help Alex deal with his problems, I was now completely overwhelmed by what was happening with Alicia, and had little energy left for him. What he really needed, during this period, was a good therapist, but he continued to resist therapy. He took his medication, and from time to time he would try therapy again, but it never lasted more than a few visits.

We got to the emergency room with Alicia around eleven P.M. She was taken right in and put on a stretcher. The cuts on her arm and wrists were superficial. A nurse washed them and put an antiseptic on them. Alicia was screaming when she arrived. She was given a sedative to quiet her. It worked for twenty minutes or so; then she began screaming wildly and trying to jump off of the stretcher. Her wrists and ankles were secured to the corners of the stretcher with thick leather straps. She lay there, with her arms and legs outstretched, screaming, thrashing from side to side, and demanding to be released. She would stop for a moment, become sad, start to whine, and then explode in another flurry of screams and efforts to free herself. A hospital security guard was posted outside her room. She was given a second dose of the sedative.

I kept thinking about David. How could he have done this? Do adolescents have no common sense, no intelligence at all? On impulse, I called him at home. "You should get down here to the hospital and see the consequence of what you've done," I told him. "You're responsible for this. Alicia's so out of control she's tied down. I want you to get over here now." He gave the phone to his mother. Fifteen minutes later, the two of them showed up at the emergency room.

I didn't know what to do next, but I couldn't sit down. I paced the hallway outside Alicia's room, trying to figure out how to fix this. The emergency room doctor examined Alicia and called for a few tests. A social worker came in to try to calm her down. When the results of the tests came back, the doctors said she was physically able to go home. Alicia said she no longer had any desire to hurt herself. "Let's get her out of here and get home," I said. It was, by now, around three A.M. I was exhausted, more from anger and worry than from lack of sleep. "I'm not sure I want to go home," she said. The emergency room doctor and the nurses were unsure what to do. If Alicia refused to go home, they would have to transfer her to the county mental hospital. It was impossible, at this hour, to try to find a bed for her at Four Winds. And, besides, it wasn't clear that she needed to be admitted to the hospital. Everything seemed suspended in time. We were getting nowhere. Liz, Matt, and David stood beside her, alternately holding her hands, stroking her forehead, and listening to her ramble on about how she felt. I lost it. I went over to the bed. "You're drunk!" I shouted. "This is your own fault. Don't tell me about your troubles. You're drunk, and if you feel like shit, it's your own damn fault!"

She screamed again, and lost control, struggling against the restraints. Liz and Matt yelled at me to get out of the room. For a minute, I thought Matt was going to try to throw me out. I was so angry, I almost wanted him to try. "I'm not coddling her any longer," I said. "She's medically checked out, she's ready to go home. I'm going home. Call me and I'll come and get you when she's ready to come home." I told them they should leave Alicia in the emergency room until she decided whether she wanted to come home or go to the hospital. Matt was furious at me. I was just as angry at him. I looked him in the eye, gave him the finger, and walked out. Half an hour later, Liz and Matt came home with Alicia. We went to bed.

No one spoke to me the next day. And I was glad to be left alone. I was still furious over Liz's and Matt's efforts to soothe Alicia, when, to my mind, she'd done a stupid thing. I thought she deserved punishment, not understanding. Now she was home, now we could figure out what to do. We had learned a couple of things at the emergency room: Alicia's psychiatrist was away on vacation. And Four Winds had no beds available for adolescent girls. The psychiatrist is always away when there's trouble, I thought. How are we supposed to know whether Alicia belongs in the hospital without checking with him?

I remember most vividly two snapshots from that night.

Alicia at home in the chair, struggling to get away from the kids holding her down, and Matt, when I looked him in the eye and gave him the finger. The reason I didn't shout "Fuck you" is that I thought one of the nurses would hear me.

These repeated angry outbursts, which I couldn't seem to avoid, were another cause for deep self-examination and recrimination. I knew they were wrong, I knew they were devastating to everyone around me, and I knew they were alienating me from my children. But I couldn't stop. Later, I began therapy myself, partly to try to understand what was happening to me. I came to realize that the anger was badly misplaced. Much of it was a product of our bitterly unhappy marriage.

The anger was meant for Liz, or maybe for myself. I was furious with myself for pretending for so long that the marriage could be salvaged. Anger arose, too, from our battles over child-rearing. I was trying to be firm with Alicia, and Liz was coddling her, I would say, over and over again. You're too strict with them, you don't yield, you don't give them a chance, Liz would reply. You set standards they could never meet. Maybe I was right, maybe she was right, maybe we were both wrong. It didn't matter. What mattered was that the pressure inside me was building, had been building for years, and I could no longer contain it. Worse than that, I kept thinking that I could contain it, that I could continue in the marriage, that I was strong, and tough, and nobody was going to make me walk away from my children. *I was going to get through this.*

As for Liz, she was coming to a similar realization. After years of conflicts over the kids, over money, over my work, over a hundred other things, Liz and I had accumulated such a weight of past hurts and unexpressed anger that the marriage could no longer support the load. The feelings we might once have had for each other had calcified into brutal disregard. We behaved badly to each other, and the kids, like Matt that night, were often caught in the middle. Even as I realized what was happening, however, I refused to admit that the marriage was over. I knew what would happen if we divorced. No matter what kind of custody arrangement we worked out, I wouldn't see the kids every night when I came home from work. I wanted to watch my kids grow up, and I wanted to keep reading and telling stories to Alicia every night at bedtime. I couldn't imagine living apart from them.

But after much reflection and thought, I recognized that it was already too late. The marriage was over.

CHAPTER SIX

When Alicia was hospitalized for the first time, in December 1999, she told the admitting doctor that "her parents fight a great deal," and that she "feels like cutting when she hears them fight." Alex had said the same thing over and over again, for four years, to psychiatrists, therapists, the school psychologist, and anybody else who asked. His parents fought all the time, he said. He was worried they would get a divorce. He was worried about his sister, who cried when they fought. Neither of them ever said much to Liz or to me. Nor did Matt, who surely would have expressed the same distress if anyone had asked him. He hadn't seen a therapist or psychiatrist, hadn't been hospitalized, and so hadn't had the chance to say how he felt about his parents' fighting.

Alex and Alicia were right. Liz and I did fight a lot. Sometimes we would shout at each other. More often, we would exchange a few cold remarks, Liz would demand a response, and I'd turn to the newspaper or a magazine and ignore her.

I was convinced that we were responsible, in part, for what was happening with the children. "Healthy parenting does not produce a self-mutilating child," the therapist Steven

Levenkron writes in *Cutting*. "If a child's experience with her parents is uncomfortable, neglectful, or painful, the child accepts the pain and assumes that her parents' behavior is justified because they must be 'right.'" As the child grows older, she relies on the parents less, and "it is then her job to re-create the pain that guided her through her early life, the pain that means home, safety, comfort." Levenkron is talking about abusive parents, who neglect their children, who are insensitive and neglectful. Surely Liz and I were not abusive parents. We loved our children, we were devoted to them, we would do anything for them. And even though we fought, we never let that interfere with our love for the children.

That's what I would have said before the children got sick. After years of therapists and psychiatrists, after telling the children's story, and our story, so many times that I could recite it by rote, I began to have a different view. When we gave the family history to a new psychiatrist or therapist, we would mention the frequent arguments as matter-of-factly as we might discuss the weather. The first few times, it was deeply embarrassing to admit that we fought as often as we did. Later, I would say it without a flicker of sadness or remorse. It was just a fact, another thing to put in the kids' medical charts, a part of their lives. It wasn't going to change. The discord was just there, in the house, like the piano, the dining room table, and the gallery of kids' pictures on the walls in the stairway: part of the family landscape.

Psychiatrists have been speculating for decades about whether bad parenting might aggravate or cause mental illness in kids. Freud and many other psychiatrists and psychologists who were prominent in the middle of the twentieth century delivered punishing verdicts to mothers, in particular. Schizophrenia was at one time believed to be caused by mothers' inappropriate behavior. Autism was blamed on "refrigerator mothers," who withheld love and acceptance from their children. They were emotionally detached, and while they could "defrost" enough to have a child, they were incapable of providing the warmth and love the child needed. Much of the latter part of the twentieth century was spent trying to extinguish these cruel and destructive stereotypes, which were the product not of research, but of armchair theorizing by, as it happened, men.

Advances in genetics helped to dispel these theories and paint a more complex picture, in which mental illness is caused by the interaction between certain genes and the environment, especially the family environment during a child's early years. During the past twenty years, researchers have deciphered the genetic underpinnings of cystic fibrosis, Duchenne's muscular dystrophy, sickle cell anemia, and many other ailments. They have so far made little progress, however, in understanding the genetics of psychiatric disorders. These illnesses are caused not by a mutation in a single gene, but by any of a number of alterations in dozens of genes. The genes interact in ways that lead to thousands of possibilities for error—and thousands of theorized causes for psychiatric ailments. Identifying all of these genes and determining how they interact will be a formidable intellectual challenge. Even that, however, will not provide a complete picture of children's mental illness. Children grow up not in sterile laboratory bubbles, but in a crowded, rich, and changing landscape of families, friends, love, hurt, disappointment, and delight. Determining how children are shaped by that landscape may be one of the toughest challenges researchers have yet had to face. No mental illness can be understood without taking genetics into account. And no mental illness can be understood without considering the role of the family, and, in particular, the role of parenting. As one researcher has put it, the development of these diseases "is 100% environment, and 100% genetic." Both are important, and it is difficult to disentangle them. "There is a constant interaction between the environment and the genetic expression of behavior," this researcher says.

Parents should therefore not be blamed for causing mental illness in their children. But they shouldn't be given a free pass, either. To put it bluntly, bad parenting almost certainly plays a role in the development of mental illness.

I began to run across research studies that underscored this idea. In one of the studies, the psychologist Jeffrey G. Johnson and his colleagues at Columbia University followed 593 parents and their children for twenty years. "Most of the youths that experienced high levels of maladaptive parenting behavior during childhood had psychiatric disorders during adolescence or early adulthood," they concluded. Maladaptive parents were those who punished their children severely, made them feel guilty, did not keep up their homes, and did not spend enough time with their children or show them enough affection. The prevalence of psychiatric disorders in adults generally is 20 percent. In the children of the maladaptive parents, the prevalence of psychiatric ailments was 63 percent.

In another study, Avshalom Caspi and a team at the Institute of Psychiatry at King's College, in London, were trying to understand the workings of a gene called 5-HTT, which, according to previous research, seemed to be related to depression. They followed a group of 847 people in New Zealand from the age of three until they were twenty-six. The researchers found that being born with a certain mutation in the 5-HTT gene could lead to depression. But the symptoms of depression and the likelihood of suicide were greater in those individuals who had a combination of two things: the gene mutation, and a stressful, difficult life, including such things as a death in the family, ill health, or mistreatment by parents. The message was that a child might be born with a predisposition to mental illness, but the family environment has a lot to do with whether the illness actually develops.

I didn't need these studies to know that the fighting that had become a fixture in our household was hurting our children. It's fair to ask whether their illnesses would have occurred at all, or perhaps have been less severe, if they'd grown up in a home with parents who cared for each other and treated one another well. We'll never know. We might not have experienced mental illness in our family if the marriage hadn't collapsed. If we'd behaved differently, we might have prevented all the suffering that our children have endured. It's something Liz and I both have to live with.

It had seemed like a good marriage for a while. During the four years before Matt was born, we had many more good times than bad. We had met working odd jobs in Boston, where we discovered that we had a lot of shared interests. We both drove Volkswagen Beetles, and we had both done a lot of traveling, hiking, and camping. We both played the piano. Liz had been something of a prodigy as a child, taking to classical piano easily and spending summers in music camps. I had started the piano a little later, progressed much more slowly, and leaned strongly toward jazz. I was in music school when we met, hoping to become a professional musician. We both enjoyed the theater. I'd done a lot of acting in high school; she'd majored in theater in college. I loved to eat fish and Liz wouldn't touch it, except for canned tuna fish with lots of mayo and onions to drown out the taste. That was about the only place we disagreed. Neither of us had much money, and that was okay by us. It is more important to do what we want and what matters, we said, than to make money. And, besides, what did we need? Not much, besides a roof over our heads. We had tents and sleeping bags. We had a guitar, on which I could bang out a few things by Dylan and Simon and Garfunkel. All we needed was money for gas, for books and records, and for a new pair of blue jeans now and then when the old ones wore out. Not when they had holes in the knees or the pockets, but when they'd become so threadbare we couldn't fix the holes.

Some things changed during those first few years. Liz found a job as a fund-raiser for a fundamentalist preacher. It was a back-office job, writing solicitations and opening envelopes, some of them stuffed with cash in small bills, probably from people who couldn't afford to be donating so much. While the preacher's target audience was mostly religious conservatives in the rural South and West, his business office was in Boston, staffed with mostly young, liberal college grads who were happy to have a reasonably well-paid job. We laughed about the Reverend, whom nobody we knew in Boston had ever heard of. Liz had gone to a couple of colleges, uncertain what she wanted to do, and had finally found a home as a theater major. But she didn't have any ambitions about going into theater professionally, so she needed to find something to do to make a living. And she was happy to have found this job. It helped get her started on a career in marketing and public relations, which she continued until the kids were born and resumed a few years afterward.

I began to do some writing on the days when I was playing piano at night, and eventually gave up the music career (at that time, I was playing three nights a week in a series of suburban Chinese restaurants) to be a writer. But we lived simply. When we took vacations, we threw the camping stuff in one of the VWs and hit the road. We rarely got on an airplane or stayed in a hotel. We didn't go out to dinner often, and when we did, it was usually at a neighborhood Mexican place, where a few bucks would get us each a large, hot plate of tacos, enchiladas, and rice and beans. We didn't feel cheated or deprived because we couldn't go to a fancier place; Mexican food was our favorite.

After a few years, we decided it was time to start a family. For the first time, we bought furniture. Our books were still shelved on planks stacked on cinder blocks, which we'd kept from college, and the rest of our furniture was hand-me-downs, things we'd found in apartments we moved into, and even a couple of items, such as my little wooden nightstand, that we'd picked up on the street on trash day. But now we needed a crib and a changing table. We spent a long time looking, until we found things that were inexpensive but looked as though they would survive a couple of kids.

I was still writing; by now I had a regular, full-time newspaper job, and I continued to freelance for newspapers and magazines and to play piano in an odd assortment of groups, usually led by an Italian singer who crooned the sentimental old favorites in American Legion and VFW halls all over greater Boston. Liz had left the Reverend and moved to a marketing and public relations position for a classical music impresario in Boston, where she had a chance to use some of what she'd learned as a theater major. The work was a lot more satisfying, and it had some cachet; we occasionally met the performers, and we often got free concert tickets.

Our income was still modest, but more than enough for me. I'm not sure Liz felt quite the same way. Her father was a doctor, a Greek immigrant who'd survived action in World War II, worked his way through medical school in Athens and the United States, and had a lucrative private practice in Connecticut when she was growing up. Liz's childhood home was a rambling eighteenth-century house on a lake, a dramatic contrast from the tiny house in which I'd grown up. She was accustomed to going on ski trips with her family; for a while, her parents owned a condominium on a ski slope in Vermont. We couldn't afford to go skiing, even if we stayed at the condominium. Liz had taken a step downward on the socioeconomic ladder, while I was perched on more or less the same rung I'd grown up on.

We first started to have little disagreements when Matt was born. We disagreed over how we should put him to bed. We had developed an elaborate feeding, cuddling, and rocking routine to persuade him to drift off to sleep. It could take half an hour, sometimes, and then if we didn't lay him in the crib gently enough, he'd wake up and we would start again. The pediatrician told us we should drop all this and let him cry himself to sleep for a couple of nights until he learned to drift off on his own, unafraid of the dark. The bedtime ritual had exhausted me, and I was ready to try anything. Liz didn't agree. She thought it would be too traumatic for him. After a week or so, I convinced her that we should try it. Matt quickly settled into the new routine, and we got over our little disagreement.

Then there was Matt's diet. Liz ate a very limited diet; Mexican food was as daring as she got. I eat almost anything, and one of the things I love about traveling is the chance to try new foods. I thought it would be great to start the kids on all kinds of different dishes, as soon as they were ready, so they would grow up liking everything. Liz didn't see any value to that, and, when Matt moved on to solid foods, it was a lot easier for her to make macaroni and cheese, or chicken fingers and frozen corn, than to whip up more adventurous things that she didn't eat. So they ate what she ate. When the opportunity arose, I'd offer the kids a bite of something different, but, most of the time, Liz made dinner while I was still at the office, and so she decided what they ate. What disturbed me was not that I was outvoted on this decision, but that I didn't seem to have a vote.

Liz quit her job just before Matt was born. We had enough money to get by without her income, for a while anyway, and we both thought it best that she be home to care for Matt full-time. But she wasn't happy. She complained that caring for the children left her exhausted. I understood that. It was a difficult job. And I had to admit that I would not have wanted to quit my job to care for the kids. I tried to help Liz as much as I could. I didn't expect to find dinner waiting when I got home. What I did expect was a little time with my wife after work. Instead, we developed a pattern in which I would relieve Liz after dinner, chatting with Matt, changing his diaper, reading him a book before bed, and putting him to sleep. Liz got a few minutes to herself. Just as I finished with Matt, she would go to bed, usually around eight or eight-thirty. The pattern continued when Alex and Alicia were born. My responsibilities for the kids ended just as Liz went to bed; then I found myself in the family room, alone. In those early years, I spent far more evenings alone than I ever had when I was single.

I was distressed by the situation. I didn't want to spend the evenings alone, but there didn't seem to be any alternative. If Liz was tired, she was entitled to go to bed. Maybe I would have done the same thing in her place. Nevertheless, it was another development that strained the ties in the marriage. I couldn't play the piano, because everyone was sleeping, so I read and listened to music instead. It wasn't that I was unhappy being by myself. As a writer, I was accustomed to spending many hours alone in front of an old Underwood typewriter (and later a computer). But Liz and I didn't seem to have much time together, not even enough to compare notes on what we'd each done that day.

At work, however, things were getting better. I'd left the newspaper for the Associated Press, where I was getting increasingly better assignments. We had moved to California for a year, and then to New Jersey, when the AP offered me a job as a science writer in New York City. I liked to bring home stories to show Liz and the kids what I'd written. Some nights, the kids would be interested, and some nights they wouldn't be. But Liz rarely was. I'd give her copies of the stories and find them, weeks later, piled somewhere, unread. I went on to write books, and she never opened one of them. I could understand the evenings alone; she was exhausted. But I couldn't understand her complete lack of interest in what, to me, was much more than a job. It hurt.

Liz began to do some temporary secretarial work after Matt was born, mostly to get out of the house and share the company of adults for a while during the day. We put Matt in day care and then in a Montessori school, and we were still breaking even, as long as I kept up the freelance writing. My AP salary didn't cover our expenses, and sometimes our money ran dangerously low, to the point where we had only a few hundred dollars in the savings account; an unexpected problem with the car, say, or the refrigerator would have wiped us out. But I was always able to hustle up a few quick assignments, and we managed to get through those years without going into debt.

When Alex and Alicia were born, Liz again stopped working for a while. Eventually, she settled into a fifteen-hour-a-week job raising private funds to supplement the Ridgewood school district's budget. Her office was only a mile from home, and she could take the kids to school in the morning and pick them up in the afternoon. She could also leave in the middle of the day if one of them got sick at school. She dropped the kids off at school, worked until noon, and then used the afternoon to run errands or relax before picking the kids up at three P.M. But she was still tired all the time, and she still went to bed too early for us to spend the evenings together. Where once we thought we had shared a lot, we now shared less and less. We rarely went to the theater; Liz was too tired on the weekends to drive the twenty-five miles into New York City. We didn't go to movies often, because of the difficulty of finding a baby-sitter. We took the kids on short hikes, but we didn't go hiking and camping the way we used to. We didn't go out to hear music. And we didn't go out to dinner anymore. I missed these things, but Liz didn't seem to. What had happened to our shared interests? Had that been some kind of illusion?

In those years, I played piano one night a week with a jazz big band. We rehearsed every week, running through old tunes by Count Basie, Duke Ellington, and Glenn Miller. We played concerts in an outdoor bandshell during the summer, for which we were not paid, and six or eight times a year somebody would hire us to play a wedding or school reunion, for which we'd each get $35 or $40. Liz brought the kids to the bandshell concerts when they were young, but as soon as they were old enough to tag along with me on their own, she stopped coming. It was years into the marriage before she told me that her expressed interest in jazz wasn't real. "I've never liked it," she said. Whenever I put on a jazz record or CD, she would ask me to take it off. If I refused, it would start an argument. From then on, I used the evenings alone to play the music that I couldn't play when Liz was awake.

As the years went on, it became unusual for the two of us to go out alone. We had less and less to say to each other. When we wanted to go out, we'd invite a group of five or six couples whom we chummed around with. It was a friendly group, and we had a good time. Liz and I sat apart. I argued politics with a couple of the men at one end of the table, and she sat at the other end, talking about something else. It was an efficient arrangement. It maintained the illusion that we could go out and have fun, while papering over the reality that we were each, separately, having fun with others in the group. We didn't embarrass ourselves by arguing in front of those friends, because we rarely talked to each other when we were with them. Whether they noticed, and whether they had a sense of some underlying difficulties, I don't know. They might well have been preoccupied with similar issues of their own.

One night, in a departure, we went out to dinner alone, to our favorite Italian restaurant in Ridgewood. The conversation languished. I didn't talk about work; Liz had little interest in what I did. And I'd long since stopped bringing her my stories. I can't remember what we talked about that night, but before long the conversation locked on to one or another of our long-standing, unresolved arguments. It could have been about the kids, about school, about turning the television on or off, about money. Whatever it was, it quickly escalated. I tried to keep my voice down. This was a small town, for God's sake; we might know somebody at one of the other tables. Just as the food arrived, Liz shouted something, stood up, and walked out. Everyone in the restaurant turned to see what had happened. I sat there alone, with two steaming, untouched plates of pasta in front of me. I stood, paid the bill, and left. I suppose I should have bowed to the other diners as I left; they had all watched the performance.

On another occasion, we were driving to see a rare local concert by a favorite folksinger of mine, Michael Smith, who was playing a few towns away in New Jersey. That time the argument was about money, as I recall. It could have had something to do with whether we were going to buy a new car or a bigger house, two moves I was opposed to, because I was already worrying about how we were going to pay for college for the kids. When I got out of the car, she got behind the wheel and said she was going home. I went into the concert hall alone. It was a Sunday night. There was no bus to get me home, and a cab, if I could find one, was going to cost $75 or $100. As it turned out, Liz had crept into the concert behind me and sat in the last row. She was waiting in the car when I came out. I was tempted to call a cab, rather than get back in the car with her. But I didn't want to spend $100 to make a point.

Our little disagreements were growing into major arguments, and eventually into colossal struggles that could never be resolved. We didn't share anything anymore. Liz was no longer interested in the piano; she rarely touched it. I'd often suggest that she meet me in New York, after work, to go to a play or a musical. She was too tired, she would say, or it was too much trouble to find a baby-sitter. The truth was, she'd lost her enthusiasm for the theater. So we rarely went. Nor did she encourage the kids to go when they were older. I'd try to get them to go, but if Mom wasn't interested, it was easy for them to say they weren't interested, either. It was difficult to camp when the children were very young. We traveled less during those years, but I looked forward to the time when we could get back to camping and hiking with the kids.

By that time, Liz had lost interest in camping. It was too much trouble to set up the tent; the ground was an uncomfortable place to sleep. When the children got older, I'd take them camping once a year on an island in the middle of Lake George, in northern New York State. Liz was happy to have that weekend at home, by herself.

We disagreed about how to spend money. I wanted to take the kids places, on trips and to museums, and into New York to wander through Central Park on a summer Sunday. We still didn't need a lot of money, as far as I was concerned—with one exception. We had to save enough to move to a town with good schools. When Matt and Alex were young, before Alicia was born, we lived in a working-class New Jersey town with mediocre schools, and I wanted desperately to move to Ridgewood, where I knew the schools were among the best in the state. And we made it; we saved, and we borrowed, and we worked our way into Ridgewood, just after Alicia was born. We struggled to make the mortgage payments the first few years. We got by with one car. We didn't travel often, and, when we did, we stayed in Comfort Inns, not Hiltons.

This was fine with me. I bought myself a few books and records, and after that I didn't want much of anything else. But Liz was increasingly unhappy with a tight budget. She wanted to fix up the house. She wanted new furniture, and she got interested in antiques. She wanted to get a second television and put it in the bedroom; I refused to allow it. She watched television frequently, I rarely did, and I didn't want the damn thing in my bedroom. I wanted to read and listen to music there.

I felt as though I was constantly putting the brakes on spending, and I grew more and more irritated about that. Liz was unhappy about it, too; she thought she deserved nice things. We lived in one of the most modest neighborhoods in Ridgewood. Many of our friends lived in bigger houses, and with their Wall Street salaries they were able to afford the kinds of furnishings that were increasingly important to Liz. I was already working two jobs: full-time as a newspaper reporter, and part-time, nights and weekends, writing free-lance magazine articles. I managed to write two books in my spare hours while I was working full-time. I enjoyed the work, but it took too much time away from the kids, and it was exhausting. And still we were only scraping by financially, and Liz was unhappy that we couldn't afford a new car, or a new sofa, or new carpeting. Once while I was away for a few weeks on a trip overseas, I came home to find that she'd bought new furniture for the family room, without saying a word to me. I didn't see how we could afford it.

Spending time with the kids was important to me. Liz felt, with some justification, that she was with them all the time, so she should get time off when I was around. I encouraged them to play sports, something I hadn't done myself. They seemed to enjoy the games, and so did I. Sometimes I missed games because of business trips, but I never missed one when I was home. Liz would go now and then, but she often stayed home. The weekends and evenings were her time off, and she had other things to do.

When I walked in the door in the evenings, after eight or ten hours at work and a three-hour round-trip commute on the train, I was exhausted. I tried to conserve whatever energy I had left for the kids. I sometimes grabbed food at the train station to hold me until I could get home, read the kids their bedtime stories, and then sit down to dinner at nine or ten. This was not a burden; even when I found my eyelids drooping and my mind wandering from what was on the page in front of me, I still enjoyed having a few quiet moments with the children. Liz rarely read to the kids.

I could see already that our arguments were having a devastating impact on Alex, Matt, and Alicia, but I didn't know how to stop. I tried not speaking to Liz at all, and not responding when she would throw out what I saw as bait for an argument. When she spoke to me, I refused to look up at her, and she'd make a crack and walk away. That wasn't much better than arguing, but at least we weren't openly shouting at one another.

In the spring of 2000, Liz and I started seeing a marriage counselor, at her suggestion. I didn't want to go. The first family therapist we'd seen had been a disaster. I had no desire to resume the tumultuous counseling sessions that had left us shouting at each other in the parking lot. I didn't think any marriage counselor had anything to offer us. We didn't get along, and that was that. But I didn't know how to say no to Liz without making it appear that I had no interest in saving the marriage. And I wanted to hold this collapsing marriage together, somehow, at least until Alicia left for college.

I knew what the consequences were if the marriage totally fell apart. I wouldn't be reading Alicia to sleep anymore, or not very often. I wouldn't be seeing any of the children as often. Despite all the suffering that our troubled marriage had put them through, I thought it was better that we stay together. More than that, however, there was a matter of principle involved. Or maybe my motive wasn't so noble; maybe it was merely pride. I had gotten myself into this marriage, and I was going to make the best of it. To abandon the marriage would be a failure, an admission that I couldn't somehow make a workable thing out of the sad situation we'd fallen into.

The sessions with the marriage counselor were unbearable. He decided early on that ours was a relationship worth saving. I don't know why he decided that. We gave him little reason to think it. I wanted only to try to maintain the status quo. If we could maintain the day-to-day business of the marriage, I'd be happy. It was a business relationship. We had kids to raise, and a budget to meet. Let's get on with it, and forget about our feelings. I didn't think we had much chance of building a better relationship. What would it be based on? How would we ever settle the unending list of disagreements? Liz did most of the talking at the sessions. I spoke when the counselor asked me to. Midway through the year, we stopped going. We were accomplishing nothing.

As our conflicts continued, I became increasingly detached from Liz, and, without realizing it, from the kids. I got up early so that I could have a little time for myself while everyone else slept, or I stayed up a little later. I tried to find a place to sit where I could read or listen to music without being disturbed. If we couldn't resolve the arguments, there wasn't much point in continuing to scrape our nerves until they were raw, day after day. It was better to simply walk around each other, avoiding interaction as much as possible.

Anger is something I've had to work on most of my life. My mother used to tell me that I had a "terrible temper" when I was young. I didn't display it often, but when I did, I regretted it. One time, when I was twelve or thirteen, I remember my father running after me across the front lawn when I'd lost control and made some angry remark. He grabbed me and sent me inside. I was terrified, because I could see how angry he was. I don't remember what either of us said or did. All I remember is the anger. That's the way it is with anger: it obliterates everything else.

When the kids were young, and the marriage was easier, I wasn't angry often. I thought the impulse to get angry had dissipated. I didn't think I had a "terrible temper" any longer. I was happy.

As Matt approached adolescence, and began to show the first signs of rebellion, flouting parental authority, I could feel the anger start to rise again. It was still there. As the marriage deteriorated, I felt it more powerfully. It became more than I could bear. It started to break out, and too often it was directed at the kids. I couldn't solve the problems in the marriage, and I couldn't do much about the children's illnesses, but I could damn well be sure that the kids behaved properly and treated their parents with a little respect. Anger colors everything, even the judgment of a father who loves his children.

It was not until I began to work on this book that I realized how much this anger was a part of me, how much it had been since I was a child. And it occurred to me that there was some parallel with Alex's illness. Anger is one of its hallmarks. Where did that anger come from? Could I have been the source of the genetic bits that gave rise to his bipolar disorder? I've never experienced the racing thoughts or the abrupt mood changes that I've seen in Alex, or that I've read about in others. I do not have bipolar disorder, but I might harbor the seeds of bipolar disorder, and I might have passed them on to Alex. My inept parenting was surely a contributor to his illness. Perhaps my genes were, too. I was quick to find fault with Liz, to blame the kids' troubles on her. But maybe much of this was my fault.

When Matt was twelve or thirteen, Liz began to wonder whether she was suffering from depression. I hadn't thought about it, but once she brought it up, I wondered, too. Maybe that was part of the explanation for what had happened to us. Depression could explain why she didn't seem capable of enjoying much of anything anymore. She went to see her primary care doctor, who, after talking to her for a few minutes, decided that indeed she was depressed, and he started her on Paxil, one of the newer class of antidepressants. A little later, Liz started seeing a therapist.

Around this time, she also began to drink more heavily, even while taking the medication. When the kids were still young, Liz would have a Bud now and then after work, or a Bud Light when she was worried about her weight. I never drank much. I joined her occasionally, but mostly I was afraid that one beer after work would be enough to put me to sleep, or at least make it difficult for me to concentrate on any work or reading I wanted to do in the evening. As the marriage soured, Liz began drinking more. The occasional beer became a beer after work every night, and then two. Some nights, it was three or four, or more. If she spoke, late in the evening, I would notice that she was slurring her words. Sometimes it was obvious; other times I thought perhaps I was imagining it. I told her I thought she was drinking too much, that a couple of beers every night was worrisome. She rejected the idea. She needed a beer or two to relax, she said, and I should stop being so goddamn uptight. I should just leave her alone. You're becoming a drunk, I said. What the hell kind of example is that for the kids? She would go upstairs to bed, leaving me fuming in the living room.

One evening in early August 2000, Liz announced that she wanted to talk to me, without the kids around. From time to time, she would decide we had to have a talk, and it invariably would have something to do with the problems in our relationship. Fine, I said. Let's talk later.

That night, she asked me to step into the backyard, to get

out of earshot of the kids. "I want a divorce," she said. "I've been working on this with my therapist, and I'm strong enough now to do it. We're both young. We have lots of good years ahead of us. We can have another life." The split would be amicable, she said. We'd divide things up fairly, we'd work things out with the kids. It didn't have to be traumatic. I hesitated. I was trying to gauge her seriousness. "Fine," I said. I went inside.

We'd been circling around this for years. When we argued, Liz would scream at me that she wanted a divorce, and I wouldn't respond. She brought up the subject only when she was angry, and I didn't take it seriously. But we both knew, as the years went on, that the marriage had burned itself out. The sessions with the marriage counselor had failed. We hadn't planned those sessions as a last chance to save the marriage, but when we stopped going, it became clear that that's what they had been. When Liz said she wanted a divorce, calmly, I still wasn't sure she meant it. But I had no energy to fight it, or even to discuss it. If that's what matters had come to, so be it. I had seen this coming, but I wanted her to be the one to ask for the divorce. Although the marriage was an empty shell, I didn't want a divorce. I didn't want to move out; I wanted to be with my kids. Maybe Liz meant it this time, maybe she didn't; but I didn't have the energy to object.

A few days later, I left for a two-week reporting trip to N'Djamena, in Chad. I'd been to Africa before, so I knew that traveling there meant confronting realities that we don't think much about at home. Questions of life and death come up routinely. It's a fascinating place, but also frightening, distant, and lonely. Nights alone in my hotel room, with a view of a crumbling wall across a weedy courtyard, and the sound of insects snapping against the screen, I thought about the marriage, and about the idea of divorce. Maybe I could gather my wits, make a supreme effort to dissuade Liz from this course, and maybe we could get to some emotional place that would be less wearing on both of us. I knew there was no chance of rekindling our bond, but I thought we might make things a little more tolerable for each other. After two weeks of thinking, I didn't know where I stood. I decided to wait until I got home to take Liz's measure once again.

When I returned home, she told me immediately that she had told Alex and Alicia that we were getting divorced. What, I said? You didn't wait until we could sit down together?

"They already knew," she said. "They could see it. They asked me, and I told them."

"That may be the most important thing we will ever have to tell them, and you didn't think I wanted to be here for it?" I said.

I don't remember whether we argued or not. To me, it was a supreme injustice. What could I possibly say to make that clear, if Liz didn't already see it? Had she done this deliberately, trying to seize the high moral ground? Or could it be possible that she didn't realize I should be part of this, that we should tell them together, carefully and thoughtfully, giving them a chance to say what they felt? Once again, I'd been left out of a critically important parenting decision.

For the next few days, she pushed me to find a mediator, urging me to get going on this. We were not going to get lawyers and go to court; we were going to negotiate. She handed me the classified section of the newspaper, with the apartment listings. The divorce had apparently been added to my to-do list. There would be no reconciliation, no chance to try to make this into some kind of workable relationship.

A couple of weeks later, Matt still didn't know. We called him at school and told him, as gently as we could, the way I'd wanted to do it with Alex and Alicia. It was a sad call.

This happened in the fall of 2000, a few months before the night when I came home to find Alicia being pinned to a chair by her friends, drunk and out of her mind. Alex had been hospitalized for the third time that spring. Matt was a sophomore at the University of Michigan. I was living in the house, as we began divorce negotiations, meeting once a week with a mediator nearby. This was supposed to be cheaper than a litigated divorce, faster, and far less acrimonious. We worked out issues regarding the children. We would have fifty–fifty custody, of course, with each of us having them for half of the week. We worked out a detailed schedule on the blackboard at the mediator's office. But what about money? We had some savings to consider, and the house, and the matter of alimony and child support.

At my urging, Liz had taken a full-time job when Matt started college. His tuition, room and board, and expenses amounted to about $30,000 a year, and I didn't think we could afford that on my salary and her part-time job, not if we wanted to have anything left over for Alex and Alicia's college educations.

I worried terribly about money. I stayed in the house that fall, while we tried to reach a settlement. I slept on the couch in the living room. We'd lived in the house for fourteen years; I had an enormous amount of work to do, packing and organizing, before I could move out. I would need a car; we still had only one. I needed a house that was within walking distance of the kids' schools, because when they were staying with me I couldn't be there to take them to school or pick them up. They would have to walk to school. I worried about our expenses, which were going to increase substantially when we began living in two households. Would we be able to afford to keep the house, to stay in Ridgewood? Or would we have to sell the house, uproot the kids, and move to a more modest community? I wanted desperately to stay in Ridgewood if we could. I thought it was important that the kids remain in familiar surroundings while their parents' marriage crumbled around them. I didn't contest Liz over the house; I thought it best that she get the place. Nevertheless, the situation was tense. The settlement negotiations didn't go well. We soon had attorneys, and what had started as mediation became a bitter dispute. It was difficult to go into a negotiation session, to be accused of cheating or deception, and then get into the same car and go back to the same house. Matt was away at college, but the atmosphere must have been almost unbearable for Alex and Alicia. I'm sure it contributed to Alicia's drunk, out-of-control evening at Christmastime. To stay in the house during those months had been a bad decision. That seems clear to me now. What was I thinking at the time? Why didn't I realize then that staying in the house could only cause the children greater pain?

I began spending more time in New York after work. I frequently went into the city on weekends to work at the office on freelance assignments. And I would stick around to go to the theater, or a movie, or to hear some jazz. Home was intolerable. We were getting divorced, the marriage was over, and I didn't have to answer to anyone about where I was, or when I was coming home, as long as I knew the kids could reach me in an emergency. It was better for all of us if I tried to stay out, I thought, until I could get my own place.

Near the end of 2000, I began seeing a woman I'd known casually for several years. I kept this to myself. No need to heat up the negotiations further by announcing that I was seeing someone. I thought I could get through the next few months quietly, conclude the negotiations, move out of the house, and then gradually introduce the kids to my new friend, and to what would become my new life.

On Saturday, December 29, 2000, the day after Alicia went into Four Winds Hospital for the second time, New York was buried in a huge snowfall. There was no question of driving the sixty miles to the hospital to see Alicia that day. But the trains were running, so I went into New York to meet the woman I'd been seeing. It was only two days after the episode in the emergency room, when I'd fought bitterly with Matt. We hadn't spoken since, and he was still seething. I'd been trying to figure out how to undo what I'd done, how to build a bridge to him and try to restore some sort of communication. But we still weren't speaking. Liz wasn't speaking to me, either, so there didn't seem much point in staying. I shoveled the snow off the driveway and the front walk, and I told Liz and Matt I was going into New York for the evening.

After I left, Liz said to Matt, "I bet he has a girlfriend in the city. He wouldn't be going into New York in this weather unless he was meeting someone." Matt used my laptop, on which I'd stored my passwords, to get into my e-mail account. He found a brief message from the woman I'd been seeing, and then got her name from my address book. He saved a copy and printed it out, and went for a long walk outside in the snow, weighing what to do. I came home late that night. Everyone was asleep. I went to bed on the living room couch.

Matt confronted me the next morning. As I was waking up, still groggy, he came into the room, leaned against the wall, crossed his arms, and asked me about the woman I was seeing. He called her by name. I couldn't immediately sort out what I was hearing. How did he know her name? I muttered something about why he wanted to know, trying to clear my mind and steady myself for what was coming.

He asked who she was.

"None of your business," I told him, slowly realizing what must have happened. "Did you look at my e-mail, you fucking prick?" We stared at each other for a few seconds.

"You were cheating on Mom!" he said.

"Bullshit," I said. "We're getting divorced, goddammit. My time is my own."

"It doesn't matter," he said. "It's wrong. You're still married." He ran to the next room to tell his mother. Liz came into the room. "Did you have sex with her?" she demanded. "Did you spend money on her?" She became hysterical. "You get out of this house right now!" she shouted. "I can't believe you would do this. Get out!"

It was a Sunday morning, New Year's Eve. Neither Liz nor I had plans that night. The next day was the holiday, so I wouldn't be able to call my attorney until Tuesday to figure out what to do. I certainly couldn't move out until Tuesday. Where would I go? I didn't know what the legal issues were, if any. Would I lose my right to make certain claims if I left the house? Could I be accused of abandoning the family?

I had tried to move out months earlier. As soon as I returned from Africa, I started to look for a place. By mid-September, I had found a house in Ridgewood. I went to see it several times, taking Alex along. I told the real-estate broker I wanted it. I was ready to walk out the door to put a few thousand dollars down, and had the checkbook in my hand, when Liz, to my surprise, told me she would not let me use money from our savings to make the down payment. I was dumbfounded. Hadn't she wanted me out of the house as quickly as possible?

She knew all about the house, and she had known for several days that I had decided to buy it. We had a huge argument. Liz's parents were there, which made the situation even more difficult. After the screaming, Liz's mother said, "Well, now we know where the bipolar disorder comes from." Meaning me. We spent the rest of the fall working with the mediator to make a deal under which I would use some of my portion of our savings for the house, but Liz would never agree. Now Liz wanted to throw me out, after she had spent four months blocking my efforts to peacefully negotiate a way out.

That Sunday, New Year's Eve, was excruciating. I tried to calm myself by playing the piano. I didn't have any relatives nearby whom I could turn to. I didn't feel as though I could show up on a friend's doorstep on New Year's Eve, and anyway, most of our friends were couples, friends of both of us. I had nowhere to go. I remember sitting at the piano, as it got closer to midnight, with Liz standing at the end of the keyboard, screaming at me to get out of the house. It was a New Year's Eve observance unlike any other.

Matt and Liz huddled during the next two days, neither saying a word to me. Later, Matt told me that Liz had started telling him intimate details concerning our married life. "I snapped at her," he said. "I told her, 'I can't be your emotional crutch all the time.'"

Later that Sunday, we drove the sixty miles to see Alicia. Matt, Liz, and I were all in one car. None of us spoke. We looked out the windows to avoid eye contact. Worried that Alicia wouldn't listen to my side of the story if Matt and Liz got to her first, I hurried in to tell her about the argument at home. Matt and Liz waited outside. Then I left Alicia while Matt and Liz talked to her. The timing of this was all wrong. Alicia was in the hospital, struggling with her depression, and it was not the time for her family to be in chaos. We spent a few more minutes with her and then drove home, trapped in the car with one another.

After our visit, the nurse on Alicia's unit noted a deterioration in her mood. "Patient was upset today but would not discuss it with the staff," the nurse wrote. Alicia "received several phone calls from family, but that seemed to upset her more." She was placed on fifteen-minute hall checks, out of concern for her safety.

That night, I asked Matt whether he wanted to talk, or whether he planned to leave things as they were. "There's nothing to talk about," he said. He left for college the next day. It was months before we spoke again.

Tuesday morning, I went to work and called my lawyer. "You need a cooling-off period," she said. "You should move out for a while." I went home that night and filled two suitcases. I left the next day for a hotel in New York. I never went back. After fourteen years in that house, I had a few hours to gather clothes and other essentials and leave. Two weeks later, I rented a house in Ridgewood, and moved the rest of my things out over the next couple of months. I never spent a night in the old house again.

It was more than a year before the divorce was final. During that year, our negotiations became even more ferocious. We had agreed to a no-fault divorce, but under New Jersey law, that meant we would have to wait eighteen months. To get things done more quickly, Liz submitted a statement charging me with unusual cruelty, which meant the divorce could be final in a few months. I didn't challenge the statement; I, too, wanted to speed the process as much as possible. I thought that would be best for the kids, and it would certainly be best for Liz and me. The negotiations were wearing us both down. Liz was still drinking, heavily enough to worry her. She had tried several times to cut down, without much success.

I grappled with consuming anger and frustration. Nothing in the negotiations seemed to be going my way. I didn't think my attorney was being tough enough, and I argued with her. I regretted hiring a woman attorney; I feared that it was easier for her to empathize with Liz's plight than with mine. At the root of the anger, however, was a central fact that I was finding impossible to bear: I had lost my children. They were angry at me over the separation, but even when that anger cooled, I spent little time with them. Teenagers are busy social creatures, and spending time with their parents is not a priority. Before the separation, I saw them every day; when they were in the mood to talk, or to ask for help with schoolwork, I was there. After the separation, we had no casual encounters. We arranged to meet for dinner. Sometimes we talked about something that was important to them, and sometimes it was just small talk. But we didn't have time together, the way we used to. That is time that I will never get back.

There is no manual for taking care of a child with a psychiatric ailment, no course at the local community college, no parenting expert on hand to offer advice. None of us is prepared for this. We all learn through our mistakes. Finding care, arranging for insurance coverage, and getting children to and from doctors' visits are the practical details that parents must work out for themselves. Working parents find themselves missing work regularly, and, when they are able to get to work, spending much of their time making calls to arrange for care. It's not unusual for a parent to quit his or her job and become a full-time advocate for an emotionally disturbed child.

Fighting with insurance companies to get reimbursement can itself consume hours every day. Relatives often withdraw from these complicated situations. Sometimes it's because they are unable to cope, and sometimes it's because they, too, blame the parents. The idea that parents caught in these circumstances might themselves need emotional support, in addition to practical help, is rarely raised.

Liz and I desperately needed help and guidance during the divorce. We needed help with the kids, and we needed help ourselves. The problems involved the entire family, including Matt, even though he was away at college. Liz was seeing a therapist. The kids had their own therapists. Nobody had a global picture of what was happening, and so all of the therapy, the medication, and the hospitalization were handled piecemeal. There was no coordination of care, and no real hope of easing the family's tensions and anxieties. We needed someone to tell us what to do, and there was no such person.

In desperation, many parents of mentally ill children have begun to turn to each other for help, through a variety of parent and patient advocacy groups. More of these groups are appearing every day. The Child and Adolescent Bipolar Foundation and the Juvenile Bipolar Research Foundation (established by the authors of *The Bipolar Child*) have undoubtedly saved the lives of many children with bipolar disorder. The first place that I found any information about bipolar disorder in children was on a parents' e-mail list run by the predecessor of the Child and Adolescent Bipolar Foundation. The depth of the sorrow and confusion that parents, mostly mothers, expressed on these lists was difficult to bear; I would read the messages for a while and then I couldn't continue. But the parents were offering one another good advice, and when professional issues arose, the foundation would seek help from psychiatrists and therapists and pass that information along to the parents on its website.

Some of these groups not only serve as resources for parents but also lobby for more research and keep a vigilant eye on all kinds of political issues that affect the families of mentally ill kids. One such organization is CHADD, which represents children (and adults) with ADHD and their families. The National Alliance for the Mentally Ill is an aggressive advocate for mental health care of all kinds, and it has a strong program focusing on children. These groups have filled a huge information gap, but they can't provide direct help to parents. That is something the health care system should be doing.

Marital difficulties are a common topic of discussion among the parents of mentally ill kids. In a nationwide survey of parents by the National Alliance for the Mentally Ill, 70 percent said their marriages had been severely stressed by caring for their sick children, and 80 percent of the parents felt that their other children without mental illness had been adversely affected by the afflicted child.

I sought a therapist with the specific goal of learning to handle the children, to control my anger, and to avoid further conflict over the divorce. I saw her weekly for almost a year. She traced much of my anger to frustration at coping with things over which I had no control. I came into her office each week complaining about what I thought was the latest outrage in the divorce battle, or some crisis with the kids, and she gave me the same response, over and over again: There is nothing you can do about that. Focus on the things you can change, not the things you can't.

My parenting skills improved, but I had little opportunity

to practice them. I had rented a three-bedroom house in Ridgewood, with the idea that we would stick to the shared custody arrangement we'd mapped out months earlier. But Alex and Alicia wanted to stay in the house they were comfortable with. My house was sparsely furnished, and it was in a different part of town, away from where most of their friends lived. I understood that it would take time for them to feel comfortable in my house, but I wanted to keep moving gradually to the point at which they would spend half of their time at my house and half at Liz's.

Even as we were breaking apart, Liz and I had one of our most consequential and damaging parental disagreements. In a surprise move, she suddenly withdrew her support of the shared custody plan. The kids didn't want to live with a father like me, she said, and who could blame them? I wasn't around much, I was too strict with them, and I couldn't give them the emotional support their mother could give them. She had decided that she would keep them at her house. Her lawyer insisted I sign a document agreeing to this. I refused. I wondered whether there was something else at work here. Liz had a strong financial incentive to seek full custody. If we shared custody, I would pay her minimal child support. If she had full custody, however, I would pay her a substantial sum each month—nearly $2,000, as it turned out. We fought over the issue for months. Alicia had a fight with her mother and spent several weeks with me, and then went back to her mother's house. Over the course of the next nine months, Alex spent no more than four or five nights at my house. I was alone there most of the time. The sight of the empty rooms depressed me. In the winter, the place was cold and drafty. I kept trying to fight for the joint custody plan; I wanted desperately to fill those rooms with my kids' sneakers, and CDs, and schoolbooks, and even piles of dirty clothes. But I could never get Liz to agree. "You are going to have to face the reality, and give up on this," my attorney said. "Shared custody is not going to happen." I didn't see what choice I had. I signed over custody of the children to Liz. I've regretted it ever since.

Liz and I don't talk at all now. We communicate only through lawyers and terse e-mails. I did not interview her for this book, although she had a chance to see a draft of the manuscript. Liz would surely tell the story of the divorce differently. But perhaps there is one point on which we could agree. The collapse of the marriage, the divorce, and the ensuing strife were disastrous for the children.

CHAPTER SEVEN

At Four Winds, Alicia began to talk about the kind of year she'd been having. We had known she was depressed, and apparently getting worse. We had watched her grades fall from As and Bs to Ds in a couple of classes, and to incompletes in the rest. Her parents' decision the previous August to divorce was noted as a "stressor" contributing to her depression. But we hadn't realized how troubled she was. She told the doctor who admitted her that she wasn't sleeping well, that she had difficulty concentrating and had a poor appetite. She had little energy, and she often thought about suicide. Shortly after she got out of the hospital the last time, she'd started drinking. She drank about twice a week, she told him, usually beer or whiskey. And she'd tried marijuana, though she wasn't a regular user.

The insurance company approved six days in the hospital: six days to undo a year's worth of suicidal thoughts and cutting. The slide into this dangerous territory occurred while she'd been seeing a psychiatrist. If he couldn't stop it while it was happening, working with her over the course of a year, what could the hospital do in less than a week? Medicate her, get rid of the suicidal thoughts, and get her out. The suicide risk was the key: once that had passed, the insurance company could argue that it no longer had to pay for hospitalization. And who but Alicia could say whether she was feeling suicidal? It doesn't take long for a thirteen-year-old who wants desperately to get out of the hospital to figure out what she needs to do: tell the doctors you no longer feel like killing yourself, and you're out. Alicia did precisely that a few days after she entered the hospital. It was impossible to know whether she meant it, but the insurance company didn't concern itself with such subtleties. When the suicidal ideation goes, so does the patient, out of the hospital and back home. "Patient denies suicidal and homicidal ideation" is how it's put in the medical chart. The denial of homicidal ideation, in a patient who has never given any indication of being homicidal, is presumably thrown in to cover all eventualities. If the patient kills herself later, the insurance company, the hospital, the doctors, the nurses, and the insurance company's lawyers can all point to the medical records showing that she no longer had suicidal thoughts. If she kills someone else, they're covered there, too. Whatever might happen, they can't be blamed.

Alicia entered the hospital on the Friday of a holiday weekend. The next three days were weekend days, when many of the regular programs, including the regular therapy sessions, were suspended. The hospital would provide individual therapy and group therapy on Tuesday and Wednesday, and she was due to be released on Thursday. That would be the six preapproved days, but the hospital didn't have all of those days to turn the situation around. Taking the holiday weekend into account, it actually had two full days and part of another.

On the Thursday that Alicia was supposed to be discharged, the nurses said they'd encouraged her to talk about her feelings in her group therapy sessions. But they reported little progress, noting that she showed few emotions, displaying "flat affect." That might help to get her a little more time in the hospital. The hospital called the insurance company and explained the situation. The insurance company granted her one more day.

A day later, her therapist wrote, "Alicia has achieved all the goals for her inpatient treatment. She has identified and practiced self-coping skills for self-harm ideation and for depression." The therapist seemed competent. She had connected with Alicia, and Alicia respected her. The nurses and the rest of the hospital staff were caring people who seemed to like the work they did. But what had they done? How did Alicia go from "flat affect" one day, to achieving "all the goals for her impatient treatment" only one day later? Operating under the constraints of the insurance reimbursements, the hospital staff set vague goals that Alicia could be said to have met after a few days. They recorded that she'd met those goals, and they let her go.

With the help of Alicia's therapist, we negotiated a contract that would spell out rules for Alicia. We asked Alicia to sign it. Liz and I signed it, too. Among the things it made clear were the specific limits that would be in place at home, and the consequences if Alicia exceeded them. The contract also made some demands of Liz and me. Among other things, it called for us to be consistent and fair with Alicia.

Alicia would be home by three-thirty on school days, unless prearranged activities were scheduled, the contract said. She would have a ten P.M. curfew. She could visit friends' houses only when their parents were at home, a reasonable precaution for a child who had admitted to regular drinking and occasional drug use. Drinking and drug use would result in being grounded for three days, and perhaps readmission to the hospital. If she lied, she'd lose phone privileges for three days. She would clean her room once a week, and she could have one friend at a time over after school. Liz and I would treat her with respect. There would be no "cursing."

The consequences of violating the contract were severe. Alicia's therapist explained that if Alicia used drugs or alcohol repeatedly, she would be sent to an inpatient substance abuse program. If she refused to follow the rules for curfew, sobriety, and going to school, she would be subject to a petition for help from the family court. A youth officer would be assigned to her, and she could be ordered into residential custody in a state institution.

Setting firm, consistent limits was something we'd been told to do a hundred or a thousand times. Long before the children became seriously ill and were hospitalized, we were told to set limits. This became another major disagreement between Liz and me, and it had festered for years. The idea of setting consistent limits and expectations, with clear rationales, was something I'd had to learn over the years. It wasn't something I recognized intuitively as a good thing. When the kids were young, I wasn't able to behave consistently and thoughtfully. When they misbehaved or had problems in school or with friends, I often didn't know what to do. Each time something happened, I'd try quickly to devise appropriate punishment and then apply it, sometimes calmly, sometimes angrily. But I came up with a different strategy every time. Sometimes the punishment was severe, sometimes mild, and sometimes I wouldn't do anything because I couldn't decide. This inconsistency in the treatment of the kids was, unfortunately, a characteristic Liz and I shared.

As the years went on, and especially when Alex and Alicia entered the hospital, I began to understand that this wasn't the way to operate. The hospitalizations were the clearest demonstration of what we should have been doing at home. In the hospital, the kids were subject to strict rules and limits, with no exceptions. They didn't like the rules, but they mostly understood why the rules were in place, and, more important, they knew exactly how they were supposed to behave and what to expect if they behaved differently. At home, we could have created a less austere version of the same thing, a set of goals, limits, and expectations that they could follow with some reasonable expectation of consistency. When Alex and Alicia were in the hospital, they seemed to thrive on the limits. The one thing that their repeated, too-short hospitalizations accomplished was to demonstrate the value of consistent limit setting. This was especially true when they were in the midst of emotional upheaval. They could cope better if they understood the rules they were supposed to follow. In the hospital, clear and consistent rule setting calmed them down.

As I realized the value of consistency, I tried to work with Liz to establish it at home. My record was far from perfect, but I felt I was learning, and I was trying to get better. Liz, on the other hand, found it difficult to acknowledge the value of setting consistent limits. As a consequence, we were never able to establish consistent rules at home. Worse, we were scarcely able to set limits at all. I tried to establish rules governing when the kids should be home at night, and requiring that they call us to let us know where they were. When they were out too late or didn't say where they were going, I'd get mad and try to apply some sort of sanction. Liz didn't think that was the way to raise children, even children with problems like ours. Her parents had used a much lighter touch, and everyone in her family had turned out fine, she said. There was no need for all the conflict that tougher standards would undoubtedly generate. And she argued that I was inconsistent. If Matt stayed out too late, he got a gentle reprimand. With Alex or Alicia I was more likely to hand out serious punishment for the same offense. I was trying to establish a consistent set of rules, but I wasn't very successful. We never did establish a consistent response. The issue became another source of arguments.

Nevertheless, we all signed Alicia's contract, which I thought was a fairly gentle document, considering the episode that had put her in the hospital. We were supposed to review it in two months, and to consider easing some of the rules if Alicia behaved well. The thing didn't last for a week. When Alicia was staying at Liz's house, Liz didn't enforce the after-school rules, or the rules about parents being home at friends' houses, or any of it. She didn't believe in the contract from the start, and she said she was too exhausted to enforce it. When I tried to enforce the rules at my house, Alicia left for her mother's house. Alicia resisted every effort we made to try to establish rules for her behavior. Liz said she couldn't take the constant arguments. Just stick to the contract, I said, with no deviation. The arguments will fade when she sees we're serious. But we couldn't do it. If we had stuck to the contract, maybe Alicia would have, too. It was a missed opportunity.

Alicia was discharged on a Friday. She was scheduled to begin a day treatment program the following Tuesday at Hackensack Hospital, which was a fifteen-minute drive from Ridgewood, much closer than Four Winds. It was the same kind of program that Alex had attended. Such programs are a way of continuing care like what children receive in the hospital, but at far lower cost. Insurance companies that balk at additional days in the hospital—that is to say, all insurance companies—are often willing to pay the far lower costs of a day treatment program, at least for a while.

Alicia's time at Hackensack Hospital was cut short, however, about three weeks after she began. The hospital called
Liz in the middle of the day to say that Alicia was being
dropped from the program and had to be picked up immediately. She had met a boy there, one of the other patients, and
had asked him for a handful of his Zoloft tablets, which she
thought would get her high, she said later. He told her he
would bring in a bottle of Zoloft from home, and give her as
many as she wanted. The next day, he tried to hand her the
pills under the desks where they were sitting. They were
caught, and Alicia was immediately taken to the office and
dismissed from the program. I didn't hear what happened to
the boy. Illicit drug use was strictly against the rules at the
day treatment program, as Alicia knew. The hospital was not
equipped to deal with drug or alcohol problems. There were
no exceptions, and no second chances. What was remarkable
about the hospital's handling of the situation is that no one
on staff there made any effort to refer Alicia or the boy to a
drug-treatment program. Would it not have made more
sense for the hospital to arrange to transfer these kids, with
their parents' permission, to another program, than to throw
them out of the health care system altogether? The dismis-
sive approach seemed to leave the kids on their own with a
difficult choice: clean up your drug use yourself, without
help, or face the only remaining alternative, the juvenile justice system. Juvenile detention centers are full of kids who
were thrown out of treatment programs.

While all this was happening, I was completely preoccupied with the sudden separation, getting out of the hotel in
New York and finding a place to live in Ridgewood. I needed
to buy a car. I needed to get more of my clothes out of the
house, and pack up my things. I had thought that setting up
a new life in a new place would be something I would plan

carefully before moving out, but there was no time for any planning. I couldn't continue living in a hotel and driving a rented car; we couldn't afford it. Suddenly all the attempts we'd made to conserve our money seemed pointless.

Now, on top of all of this, Alicia was falling apart. The hospitalization had been a failure. She'd been thrown out of the day treatment program. The day after that, she was read-mitted to Four Winds. The "precipitant" for her readmission, the hospital noted, "appears to be the parents' recent separa-tion."

Alicia said she hadn't had the impulse to cut herself, and she hadn't done it recently. There was no evidence of recent cutting on her arms. But later that night, after Alicia had been taken to her hospital room, she started cutting herself again. She asked another patient to notify the staff, and she started crying. She was not herself. When a couple of mem-bers of the staff came up to quiet her, she lost control, push-ing them out of the way and trying to run. They held her down while she screamed for them to let her go. As soon as they could hold her still, they gave her a PRN, an injection of a quick-acting sedative in the hip. It didn't take effect imme-diately, so they pinned her arms and took her to the quiet room, called the annex. The staff couldn't find anything on her that she might have used to cut herself. All the sharps, the obvious things such as scissors, nail clippers, and shavers, were, of course, locked up. Alicia told the staff she cut her-self with a piece of paper. She was kept in the quiet room overnight, until she could be reassessed in the morning. The next day, she told one of the social workers she was feeling suicidal again, and that she once again felt the urge to cut herself.

Liz and I visited separately every day. Alicia seemed happy to see me. I was now accustomed to an odd feeling of closeness with Alicia and Alex when they were in the hospital. It was during the times when they were most upset, so much so that that they needed to be confined to be kept safe, that they were most affectionate and open with me. Alicia and I talked about what had been going on, with the divorce and separation. I tried to follow her lead, to talk about the things she wanted to talk about, and not to push her where she didn't want to go. I didn't criticize her mother or say anything about the divorce or separation beyond what she asked. But she continued to feel depressed. The hospital psychiatrist decided to try switching her from Paxil to Effexor, to see whether it might be more effective in easing the depression.

The reasons for medication changes like this were always a little unclear. I looked into the existing research on antidepressants and discovered that little is known about the effectiveness or the best use of antidepressants in children. And there is no research comparing one drug to another. Psychiatrists who deal with kids regularly develop hunches. They get a feeling that one antidepressant might work better than another in a given kid who reminds them of others for whom, say, Effexor worked. But hunches can be wrong; it's impossible to evaluate the effectiveness of drugs without a rigorous study, comparing one drug to another or to a placebo, in two similar groups of patients. Some psychiatrists are quite skilled at using drugs, despite the lack of clear scientific guidance. But I wonder how much their feelings and hunches about certain drugs are colored by information a drug company might have sent them or presented at a medical meeting. When new antidepressants are put on the market, they often quickly replace existing, older antidepressants. Is that because the new drugs have been proven better than the older drugs? No; new drugs are tested against placebos, not against existing drugs. No one knows whether the new drugs are better. The reason new drugs take off is because they are backed by multimillion-dollar marketing and advertising campaigns. In nearly every case, the new drugs cost more, and earn more money for the drug company, than older drugs. The deciding factor in whether to switch kids from one drug to another ought to be based solely on whether the new drug is likely to work better, not on a drug company's balance sheet or marketing plans. But drug companies have no incentive to test one drug against another; what if the older, cheaper drug turns out to work better? And the government, with rare exceptions, does not require such testing.

Maybe the Effexor helped Alicia more than Paxil had; I couldn't tell, and I don't think anyone else could either. Alicia's urges to cut herself persisted. Her therapist scheduled a family session, and Alicia cut herself immediately before it. In a meeting with us before bringing Alicia into the room, the therapist urged us to stop arguing in front of the children. "These marital arguments must stop now," the therapist said. "They are damaging Alicia. You cannot argue in front of her."

It seemed an obvious point, but we could not comply. For all my failings as a parent, I did understand that when Liz and I disagreed over something, we needed to have that discussion, or argument, out of earshot of the children. They would, of course, feel the tension, and they would know that all was not well, but they would at least be spared the pain of hearing every verbal blow that we inflicted upon each other. For years, I had tried to establish ground rules under which we would step outside to do battle. Ours was a small house, and there was no place indoors where raised voices wouldn't be heard all over. I blamed Liz, but the truth is that I'd broken the rule often enough myself, sometimes unable to keep myself from letting the words fly. It had been the same for years; the children heard far more of this kind of talk than they should have.

It was also essential, the therapist said, that we did not try to bring Alicia into the arguments by criticizing each other in front of her. That, at least, was something I had scrupulously avoided. As someone who by now thought of himself as a failed, inept parent, I tried to stick to the few things I knew were right.

After that conversation, Alicia joined us. We talked about the arguments, and we said we would try to do something about them, but I doubt we were very convincing. At the end of the session, Alicia surprised me by saying she wanted to live with me, rather than her mother, when she got out of the hospital.

Alicia was sent to the quiet room that night, so the staff could keep a close eye on her and prevent any further cutting. She had a bag with her containing some of her belongings. When the staff searched it, they found a razor in the bottom. Alicia had undergone a body search, and everything she had brought into the hospital with her had been searched. But the staff had missed razor blades tucked inside her bra.

She was kept in the quiet room the next day. She told the staff she felt better; the urges to cut had subsided. Later that day, she went back to her room, but she was checked every fifteen minutes. By the next day, she was on a self-check system, reporting to the nurses' station every fifteen minutes on her own initiative. She looked brighter and said she felt brighter. She was encouraged to seek out a staff member for a one-on-one conversation if she felt the urge to cut herself again.

During the next few days, Alicia's depression seemed to

ease. The switch from Paxil to Effexor might have been part
of the reason. Or maybe it was therapy, or maybe the environment in the hospital, with its clear, rigorously enforced
rules. She told the staff she felt that she would do much better upon her release from the hospital this time. She wasn't
quite ready to declare that she would no longer drink or
smoke marijuana when she got out, but she was beginning
to admit that doing so was harmful. The psychiatrist added
Risperdal, an antipsychotic, to her medication regimen, to
try to deal with her mood swings and occasional irritability.
Risperdal, like most psychiatric drugs, hasn't been tested in
children, but it is widely prescribed to calm them down.

After seven days in the hospital, Alicia had shown distinct
improvement. But her therapist and psychiatrist were still
concerned enough about her safety to continue requiring
safety checks every fifteen minutes. That suggested she
might still cut herself or entertain suicidal thoughts. Alicia
had a long way to go, I thought, if she needed to be checked
every fifteen minutes. That apparently didn't trouble the
insurance company, however. She was discharged the next
day. The patient "denies SI/HI" (suicidal ideation, and homicidal ideation), her records show.

The records also show that she "expressed a commit-
ment to refrain from substance abuse upon discharge." It was
a foxhole conversion. The day before, she hadn't been so
sure. Now that she had the opportunity to leave, she was
happy to renounce drug use.

The plan was that Alicia would return to school, see her
psychiatrist regularly and see a therapist every week, and live
with me. She'd argued with her mother, and didn't want to
stay with her. I was glad that Alicia wanted to live with me. I
looked forward to setting up a routine for the two of us. But

I was a little concerned about her motives. Did she really want to stay with me, or was she trying to send some message to her mother?

I was concerned about whether I'd be able to supervise her properly. Her counselor at the middle school recommended that we send Alicia to a school for emotionally disturbed kids. Alicia was not ready to return to the rigors of the public school, the counselor believed, or to the company of the girls who had turned on her not so long ago. Alicia pleaded with us to return to the middle school. She persuaded me that she could handle it, and I argued her case with the counselor. We made arrangements to have her picked up at my house, and brought back there after school. She was to stay home then, doing her schoolwork. I told Alicia that she could not have friends over while no adult was home, but that I'd be willing to relax that rule later on if she did well. I arranged my work schedule so that I would work from home one day a week, and get home earlier in the evening every day except for one, when I had late deadlines to meet.

The arrangement lasted about two weeks, until my parents came to Ridgewood for a visit, something they did once or twice a year. Alicia protested that she couldn't have dinner with them on a Friday night, because she had things to do with her friends. "You can do things with your friends on any Friday night," I told her. "Your grandparents are here this weekend, and you're having dinner with us." We went to a restaurant. When we got there, Alicia said she was going to call her mother to come and pick her up. "You are not going to call your mother," I said. "You are going to sit here and eat your dinner." I was trying to avoid a situation in which every time she was unhappy with me, she called her mother. Likewise, I didn't want her to call me when she was with her mother. We couldn't let her play us off against each other. "You can't keep me from calling Mom!" she shouted. "You sit down," I said. By now, everyone in the restaurant was aware of what was going on. Just as the food arrived, we got up and left. When we got home, I took Alicia upstairs and told her to stay there. The next day, I discovered that she had cut herself deeply several times on her left shoulder before she went to bed. That weekend, she moved back to her mother's house.

From time to time, she came over for dinner, or stayed for a sleepover with a couple of friends. But she didn't live at my house again. This time, I wasn't sure what had gone wrong. I'd made what I thought was a reasonable demand, that she have dinner with her grandparents, and I'd refused to yield to her complaints. Once again, I was trying to establish some limits for her behavior. This was a new situation for me. I was trying to figure out how to be a single parent. I needed some time to get it right, But I didn't get that time. A little more than a month after the separation, I was living alone in a three-bedroom house. Matt was still not speaking to me; he stayed with his mother when he came home from college in the spring. He spent the summer at school—to avoid me, he said later. Alex and I were not speaking, either. He, too, was grappling with the strains of the separation. Like Matt, he blamed me for "cheating" on his mother. He came to the house even less often than Alicia did.

I had insisted that Alicia come home after school and stay there, alone, until I got home. Liz would let Alicia visit friends, and have friends over during those perilous after-school hours, when few parents are home and almost anything can happen. We'd had a meeting with her counselor and others at the school to discuss this very issue. Liz and I sat at a table with Alicia's child-study team, four or five teachers and counselors. Each of them, in turn, said that it was critical to provide after-school supervision for a child who had used drugs and alcohol, and cut herself, and had repeatedly tried to commit suicide. The principal said he could get her a job as an after-school counselor at the day-care center at the YMCA. She could walk there after school, and she would be busy until I got home and picked her up. It sounded perfect. A few days later, Alicia said she didn't want the job.

Now that we lived separately, Alicia could choose to live with me and endure what I thought were reasonable limits. Or she could live with her mother and avoid many of them. What kind of choice was that? What teenager would choose to live with the more restrictive parent?

By the spring of 2001, several months after I had moved out of the house, the situation was worse than I could have imagined when Liz and I decided to divorce. I'd expected to see the kids half the time, instead of every day. And I knew the process would be difficult, but I figured we would work it out. Now I rarely saw the children. When we did see each other, it was tense, and difficult. I knew I hadn't been a particularly good parent, but I'd tried to be. Couldn't they see that? I loved them, and I liked spending time with them, and now I'd lost them, all three of them. None of them would ever live in my house again.

Another secret Alicia confided only to her journals was a preoccupation with her weight. This had developed during the time in and out of Four Winds, in January. For the next few months, she dabbled in anorexia and bulimia. She would stand in front of the mirror, examining what she thought was the fat that had to go. No one could have suspected that Alicia was concerned about her weight. She had a near perfect figure. "Look at the fat ooze over my jeans," she wrote. "I must punish myself for this." And, a few pages later: "The thing that David hates most is fat girls." In large letters on another page, she wrote, ALICIA = FAT.

Anorexia and cutting are both forms of self-mutilation, so it wasn't a complete surprise to learn that Alicia had developed an unhealthy image of her body. She also, in one journal entry, mentioned burning her own palm a couple of times, simply to feel the pain. I understood at the time that she could develop an eating disorder, and I kept watch, but I saw no signs of it. Anorexia is not easy to hide. While it might have been possible for Alicia to conceal how much she was eating, and to sneak into the bathroom to throw up without anyone noticing, eventually the effects would have become obvious.

In Four Winds at the end of January, she stopped eating, except at dinner, when she tried to eat as little as possible. There is no mention of this in her hospital records; none of the staff members caught on. "I've lost 4 pounds so far, but I wanna lose 16 more," she wrote. Fortunately, the idea soon lost its appeal. After a few months, perhaps as a result of her treatment and therapy, perhaps not, Alicia lost the obsessive concern with her weight. She stopped throwing up after eating, and she resumed a normal diet. She did lose a little weight, but not because she had tried to avoid eating. "God knows how that happened, but whatever. Good news," she wrote.

It was now Alicia's turn to repeat Alex's experience of shifting diagnoses. Until now, she had been thought to have major depression. But as it became clear that the sexual assault was still interfering with her efforts to steady herself, her psychiatrist decided that maybe something else was going on. He began to suspect dissociative disorder.

I asked him what that was. Think about how your mind wanders when you're driving, he said, and you suddenly realize you've missed an exit. Or you just put your car keys down but can't remember where. That's dissociation. We all do it, and in most cases, it's normal. But when it becomes severe, it can leave people disconnected from others and from their surroundings, with a sense of unreality. And it often follows severe life-threatening trauma, such as a sexual assault.

This diagnosis, too, seemed to fit Alicia. The psychiatrist suggested that we have her undergo a special, three-hour interview to confirm it. He helped us to find a psychologist who could do the test, which would cost $500 to $1,000, depending upon the time it took. Alicia did have dissociative disorder, according to the psychologist: "She has severe depersonalization—a disconnection from self. When she has her cutting experiences, she feels she can't stop." Alicia was also suffering from severe "derealization," which the psychologist said was a feeling of "going through the motions, that everything around her was fake." And she had severe "identity alteration," meaning that she sometimes "acts like a different person and that there are different sides of herself." All this was a direct result of the trauma Alicia had experienced. "It's very important that you know you have a normal, healthy girl in every other way," the psychologist said.

I suppose that last comment was meant to be reassuring. It didn't surprise me that Alicia had been traumatized by the rape; she had been working with various therapists for some time to learn to recover from that. We had a new diagnosis, but what were its implications? And it was a little too pat: "dissociative disorder" explained everything that had happened. Later, when I read the records of Alicia's psychiatrist, the diagnosis of dissociative disorder had disappeared. Not long after Alicia had undergone the interview with the psychologist, her psychiatrist concluded instead that she was suffering from a combination of posttraumatic stress disorder and anxiety. "Dissociative disorder" had been another blind alley.

It remained dramatically clear, however, that something was wrong. In April, during Alicia's spring break, she and I decided to spend a few days as tourists in Boston, visiting the museums, Faneuil Market, the bookshops around Harvard Square, and the restaurants in Little Italy. It was a happy, carefree time. We walked all over Boston and Cambridge, up and down Beacon Hill, through downtown and the Back Bay, and from MIT to Harvard and back again. It was the first time in many, many months that we had been able to spend some time together free from concerns about school, hospitals, psychiatrists, medication, and the divorce. Each night, however, when we returned to our room in a hotel on the Charles River, I noticed a curious and disturbing phenomenon. Alicia would leave the room to have a cigarette outside the hotel's front door, and then come back upstairs, lie down on the bed, grab the remote, and turn on the television. We tried to find old movies, or watched reruns of old TV shows on Nickelodeon. As soon as Alicia began to relax, however, her mood plummeted. I could see it happen. In the space of fifteen minutes, no more than that, she sank into the bed, her head drooped, her face darkened, and the light in her eyes dimmed. She was nearly immobilized, unable to speak, and barely able to respond to my questions about whether she was okay. This happened each of the three nights in Boston. And each morning she was fine again.

She was taking antidepressants at the time, but it seemed obvious that they were not working too well. I wondered how often she suffered these sudden deflations in mood when she was home, and what she might do while in that disturbing state of mind. I told her psychiatrist about it, but I couldn't tell how he received the information. He didn't seem surprised.

Three months later, on May 15, Alicia swallowed a bottle of Celexa, an antidepressant that Alex had once taken. Liz was then dating the father of one of Alicia's best friends, Sarah. Earlier that night, the four of them had gone out to dinner. Alicia had seemed fine, Liz told a counselor at the emergency room. After dinner, Liz and her date took Alicia home, and then they left. Alicia found the Celexa in the medicine cabinet. She couldn't remember how many pills were in the bottle. After taking them, she called David. He called a friend of theirs, and that friend told his mother, who called 911. The police showed up at the house and called an ambulance to take Alicia to the emergency room. The police found the bottle of Celexa. In black ink, on Alicia's forearm, were the words "Alicia hates everybody." She said she'd written them earlier that evening. Liz, Sarah, and Sarah's father went to the emergency room later that night. I would have been there, too, but nobody called to tell me what was happening.

Early the next morning, Alicia was transferred by ambulance to Four Winds Hospital. It was her fourth stay there. That's when I learned about this latest suicide attempt. I had last seen Alicia the day before, when she and I had had a session with her psychiatrist.

At the hospital, the admitting doctor noted that Alicia had had a difficult month. She'd been quarreling with her boyfriend, drinking, and smoking marijuana, and she "refuses to visit her father," the doctor wrote. She was not attending school regularly and was not doing homework, so she was doing poorly in school. A few hours later, she was back in a room in the hospital, on fifteen-minute safety checks.

Within a few days, in a pattern that was now familiar, Alicia's mood had improved. She participated in hospital activities and got along well with the patients and staff. Once she was back in a structured environment, with clear, unambiguous rules, her mood improved. The psychiatrist noted that she had a "severe biological predisposition" to depression. I noted the careful use of the word "predisposition." That suggested not that Alicia was doomed to be depressed, but that, in the right environment, the predisposition might be overcome. And her behavior in the hospital seemed to be proof of it. If we could create something like that for her at home, I was sure she would do much better. But that was out of my control. Alicia was not living with me, and I had to watch, powerless, as her mother refused to institute the rules and limits that I thought were appropriate. I waited for the next suicide attempt. Sooner or later, she was going to succeed. I thought about it day and night: We were going to lose her.

A week after Alicia was admitted, she received distressing news. She would not be leaving the hospital, as she always had before, and going home. Her psychiatrist at Four Winds was making desperate calls to the insurance company to insist that it cover additional time in the hospital. He wanted enough time to find a residential treatment center for Alicia. After four hospital admissions and repeated suicide attempts, the hospital and Alicia's psychiatrist in Ridgewood had decided that she could not be discharged. Unless she was living in a facility where she could be under constant supervision, "I don't know how to keep her safe," her psychiatrist told me on the telephone. Alicia spent most of that day in her room at the hospital, crying.

The next day, Alicia argued that she was improving, that she should be allowed to go home rather than being sent to a residential treatment facility. The place the hospital was looking at was outside Philadelphia, about two hours from Ridgewood. Alicia and I were talking again; as always, our relationship improved when she was in the hospital. The days dragged on, as arrangements were being made for a placement at the residential center. Each day, the psychiatrist was on the phone with the insurance company, arguing for another day or two. Each time, the insurance company would grudgingly give its approval for one more day, or two, but refuse to extend Alicia's stay any more than that. Her mood wavered. The psychiatrist started her on Depakote, added Risperdal, and after a week, increased the doses of both. When she realized there was no longer any point in arguing, she became resigned to the idea of a residential placement.

By the time she left Four Winds, she had been in hospitals a total of thirty-two days. Alicia was covered for ninety hospital days over the course of her lifetime. At the age of fourteen, she had used one-third of her lifetime coverage. And for most of the remaining days, I would be responsible for a large share of the cost. The hospital officials were shocked. Most plans provide for a limited number of days per year, thirty perhaps, or sixty, they told me. They had never heard of a plan with a lifetime cap.

Alicia was discharged on May 30, in the afternoon and accepted for admission to the Devereux Beneto Center in Malvern, Pennsylvania. But Devereux would not be able to take Alicia until June 14. The insurance company refused to pay to keep her in the hospital until then, despite the recommendations of her psychiatrist at home and the hospital psychiatrist, both of whom feared for her safety at home. That meant Alicia would have to be watched closely for two weeks. Liz and I were both working and unable to take that time off. We arranged with friends and other parents to see that she was closely supervised, although it was impossible to maintain the hospital's routine of safety checks every fifteen minutes. Alicia was unhappy at the thought of being sent away, but she seemed to be in reasonably good spirits. We had no close calls, no suicide attempts, no angry outbursts, and no descent into depression. It was a huge relief when I put her into the car to drive her to Devereux.

The Devereux Beneto Center is located on rolling pastureland, on what was once a farm. Some of the farm buildings are still there, converted to other uses by the school. They're a little tattered and worn. The campus is orderly and well kept, but looks as if it were run by a frugal farmer, who fixes up the doors and windows when he has to but otherwise puts his money into raising crops, or, in this case, caring for children. The high-school-age residents, most of whom come from eastern Pennsylvania and New Jersey, live in small groups in four rambling houses scattered around the property, and in two houses off campus. Elsewhere on the campus are a high school, playing fields, a gym, a swimming pool, and tennis courts. Every window has a view of golden fields, and the air is fresh. Kids who have had to struggle with dark, difficult feelings can open up and breathe there.

Devereux initially expressed some hesitation about admitting Alicia, because of what had become fairly extensive drug use. Before she was admitted to the hospital in May, she had been smoking a pack of cigarettes a day and three $20 bags of marijuana a week, and getting drunk three times a week. She told Devereux she was still smoking cigarettes, but that she had stopped using drugs and alcohol when she went into the hospital, and that she felt much better as a result. She also told the Devereux psychiatrist that she had felt depressed since the second grade, years before I or anyone else had suspected it.

At Devereux, Alicia was expected to participate in therapy, do her schoolwork, and follow the rules of the house she lived in. The rules included things such as observing curfews and lights out. And they also spelled out how the students should treat one another. The students picked up points when they behaved appropriately, and they lost points when they used profane language, showed disrespect to others, or disobeyed rules. As they accumulated points, they climbed up through a series of steps offering more and more privileges. Alicia would be allowed to call home two nights per week. She could not call her friends. More use of the phone would come as she built up points for good behavior. It was a powerful motivator.

Two weeks after she arrived, Alicia had earned enough points to move to one of the off-campus houses reserved for residents with the highest point totals and the best behavior. She had initially been put in a housing unit with eleven other girls who were "highly agitated," as the school put it. She was moved to a smaller unit, with four other girls, and then to the off-campus housing. The students there were still carefully supervised, but they were subject to fewer restrictions. Her rapid progress during those first two weeks was another example of how well Alicia responded to structured, predictable rules and expectations. That alone was not going to be enough to solve all her problems, and it certainly wasn't going to alleviate her depression, but it made her much hap-

pier and removed a lot of the difficulties that were exacer-
bating her depression and her poor estimation of herself.

At first, Alicia was not allowed to visit home; she would
have to earn that privilege, though Liz and I were allowed to
visit her. Before she could visit home, we were required to
agree to a detailed plan that would spell out exactly what she
was allowed to do while home, and who she could see. The
idea was to provide careful supervision, to assure her safety.
However much she might have improved in a few weeks,
she was still in danger of harming herself or even making
another suicide attempt. After each visit, Liz and I were
required to fill out a report noting any instances in which
Alicia did not follow the agreed-upon ground rules.

Before the first visit, about a month after Alicia started at
Devereux, I raised the question of her cigarette smoking. I
had forbidden the children to smoke at my house. That was
one more reason why they preferred to stay at their
mother's. Liz had quit smoking when we got married, and
had not smoked for more than twenty years, but she started
again after we separated. And she let the kids smoke at
home. She and Alicia made cigarette runs together. When I
stopped by the house to pick Alicia up, I'd find the backyard
littered with butts. I had covered smoking for years as a
reporter, and this was a huge issue for me. I had spent years
as a teenager putting pressure on my mother to quit, which
she eventually did. As a reporter, I covered the tobacco industry in the 1980s, long before knowledge of the industry's
covert promotion of smoking to children and its manipulation of the truth had become widely known. I knew how
tobacco companies manipulated children, and I couldn't
stand to see it happening with my kids. Every day, at work, I
saw press releases about the health effects of smoking, or

some new tobacco industry court case. I was passionate about the subject, and unable to let it go, even for a while. This was another addition to the long list of issues on which Liz and I disagreed. Again, I was powerless to do anything.

What was even more frustrating was that I was unable to convince Alicia's therapist at Devereux to pay attention to it. "My personal feeling is that Alicia has a lot of things on her plate right now," the therapist told me in a telephone conversation before the first home visit. "The big behaviors she really needs to work on changing are the drinking, the cutting, and the marijuana. You should put your energy into those issues." To my mind, smoking was of a piece with these other issues. Alicia was using alcohol, drugs, and cutting to try to cope with her emotional problems. One goal of her therapy was to help her move toward safer, more productive ways to cope, dropping the injurious behaviors. To me, smoking was another injurious behavior, another unproductive way to cope. Let's move consistently toward the elimination of all unhealthy coping strategies, including smoking, I suggested. I asked, as a compromise, that we go slower with the smoking, putting only a little pressure on that now and more later on, so that she would be able to quit by the time she left Devereux. Her therapist refused. I could see the point, that the other drugs and the cutting were immediate problems, requiring immediate solution. The damages from smoking would come decades later. But the risk that Alicia might attempt suicide again now seemed small. Smoking was emerging as a greater risk, and I could not give up on it. I couldn't put out of my mind a vision of Alicia getting better after a long, difficult, and courageous struggle, leading a productive life, and then being cut down in her fifties by a stroke or a heart attack, a consequence of smoking. Wasn't her physical health as important as her mental health? It was an argument I could not win. Alicia is still a smoker.

Before approving a home visit, her therapist insisted that Liz and I structure Alicia's time while she was home. "Activities need to be planned, so she doesn't have a lot of downtime," she said. I had to make sure there were no sharp objects in her bedroom. If she was going to see friends, they had to come to her house, where she could be supervised. "She needs to prove she's going to be responsible and follow the rules," her therapist said. "Maybe next time she can go out for an hour."

As Alicia's first home visits began, in July and August, she saw her friends only briefly. She didn't seem as eager to spend time with them as I'd expected her to be. I took that as a sign that she was developing some distance from some of the kids she'd been with when she was using drugs and drinking, as I assumed, most of them did. I didn't know them; these were the friends she had hung around with in town, after school, unsupervised. They went to houses where the parents weren't home, the houses of families I didn't know. Liz gave Alicia a cell phone after we separated, so Alicia felt no need to call to say where she was going. "You can reach me any time you want on my cell," she said. Because Alicia had been living with her mother, I didn't know whom she had been spending time with, nor did I know whether Liz had tried to keep Alicia away from the kids we suspected were drug users. Not that it was easy to tell who they were. The only sure sign was that one of them would occasionally disappear into rehab for a few weeks or months. And when these kids returned, who knew whether they were staying off drugs, or going right back to them?

The first weekend she was home, Alicia talked to the woman who had come to the house to tell me that Alicia had been raped and the police had been called. This woman, the mother of one of Alicia's friends, had had a difficult childhood herself. She had taken an interest in helping troubled kids, including Alicia. Before Alicia went to Devereux, she had spent more time at this woman's house than anywhere else. There was always a group of kids there, many of whom I didn't know. I worried about whether Alicia was being appropriately supervised there, but she was living with Liz then, and all I could do was express my concern. Alicia felt she could talk to this woman more easily than to any other adult. I hoped that was a good thing, but I couldn't be sure what to think about this relationship.

During that first visit home from Devereux, Alicia was not allowed to go to the woman's house, but the woman said she and her son, and a few other friends of Alicia's, would come over to my house to see Alicia on that Saturday night. We went to the store, bought some snacks and sodas, and waited. We watched TV, and we watched the time. By nine-thirty or ten, when it seemed clear nobody was coming, Alicia started to cry. The woman and her son never showed up. We opened a bag of chips, sat on the couch, watched a movie on TV, and tried to salvage the evening. I could understand this behavior coming from teenagers. But what had this woman been thinking? How could she disappoint Alicia like that? It was the end of Alicia's relationship with her. Although I ached for Alicia that night, I was happy to see the woman out of the picture.

During the months at Devereux, Alicia said she lost the impulse to cut herself to relieve stress. The suicidal thoughts faded away. She was relaxed and happy. She was earning near the maximum of available points for her behavior at school, sometimes earning bonus points that put her over the theoretical maximum. She began to argue that she should be discharged. She was ready to come back to Ridgewood, and back to Ridgewood High School. Her classmates had moved there without her that September, and she wanted to join them. Every two weeks, she and I had a family therapy session by telephone, with Alicia in her therapist's office, on the speaker phone. (She had separate sessions with Liz.) Alicia took advantage of the sessions to say that I wasn't listening to her the way I should, and that I hadn't given her proper credit for her efforts to pull herself back from the brink of depression and suicide. I agreed, and told her I would try to be more aware of that in the future. I raised questions about rules for behavior when she got home, and she agreed that she couldn't go on as she had, resisting any attempt to structure her time. We had one of those sessions on the morning of September 11, 2001, just after the attack on the World Trade Center, which was visible from *BusinessWeek*'s offices. The two towers collapsed while we were on the phone. Awareness of that catastrophe would hit me later; at that time, nothing, not even the destruction of the World Trade Center, seemed more important than that phone call with Alicia.

In the fall, Alicia's therapist at Devereux began to talk about a December discharge. This seemed too soon to me. While I felt good about Alicia's progress, I wasn't convinced that she was strong enough yet to resist slipping back into old habits and into depression. When she returned to Ridgewood, she would need to deal, once again, with the issues surrounding the divorce. She might resume seeing David, who had given her the alcohol that had sent her to the hospital the previous December. She would be back in school with some of the same kids who had driven her to desperation a few years earlier. And she would be associating with the friends with whom she had consumed so much alcohol and so many drugs before entering the hospital. There was no way to keep her away from them; drinking, marijuana, and harder drugs were ubiquitous in Ridgewood.

I was, however, eager for Alicia to return to regular schooling. The instruction at Devereux was far below the level at which she could have been working. I was concerned that the more time she missed, the harder it would be for her to cope with the rigors of the Ridgewood schools.

Alicia had attended meetings of Alcoholics Anonymous at Devereux, and she agreed to continue in AA when she returned home. She also said that she would submit to random urine screens.

She was discharged from Devereux on December 21, in time to spend Christmas at home and begin classes at Ridgewood High School after New Year's Day. She went to a few AA meetings after she got home. For a while, attendance at AA meetings became a social activity for Alicia and a friend. In one brief, uncomfortable visit that Liz had insisted on with my parents, she told them about the great strides she was making in dealing with her own drinking. She said she was thinking of going back to school to prepare for a career as a counselor, to try to help others.

When Alicia got back from Devereux, her friendship with Sarah began to change, as friendships among teenage girls often do. Alicia no longer considered Sarah a best friend. Yet they were together all the time, because Liz and Sarah's father were together all the time. After a while, Alicia stopped going to the AA meetings with her friend. Liz and Sarah's father stopped dating a few months later, and Liz stopped going to meetings, too. Liz didn't insist on the periodic urine screens that Alicia was supposed to undergo, and they were not done.

Around the time that Alicia left Devereux, we heard from

Four Winds Hospital. The fight over insurance coverage for those extra days had not ended the way we thought it had. Because of worries about Alicia's suicide attempts, her hospital psychiatrist had worked hard to get coverage for an extended stay of two and a half weeks. It had been an almost daily struggle, but the insurance company had grudgingly acquiesced. Months later, the hospital notified us that the insurance company had made a mistake. Those extra days were fully covered, we thought at the time. The insurance company had told me, a couple of years earlier when Alex was hospitalized, that it would provide full hospital coverage for only fifteen days, and after that the coverage would drop to 70 percent. But during Alicia's stay it had assured us that she was covered. Upon further examination, however, the insurer decided that it had been right the first time. It was required to pay only 70 percent of Alicia's hospital costs after the first fifteen days. It might seem reasonable that the insurance company should honor what it had told us, that it should cover the whole bill, because it had made a mistake. But that's not what happened. The company reduced the payment it sent to Four Winds, and we were responsible for the balance. Six months after Alicia's discharge, we got a bill for $1,898. Please pay up, the hospital said. We had no choice.

During the years when Alex and Alicia were being treated for their illnesses, we were covered by a more-or-less typical corporate health insurance plan provided by my employer. I paid extra for a plan that covered not only doctors on the list of preferred providers, but also those outside the plan's network, who were, of course, covered at a lower rate. It was never entirely clear how much lower that rate would be, however. Psychiatrist No. 7 refused to accept any health insurance reimbursements. Like a growing number of psychiatrists, who are themselves fed up with the health care system, he required payment up front, at the rate of $275 per hour. This was supposed to be reimbursed by the insurance company at some rate lower than 100 percent. Exactly how much the insurance company would pay for these visits was based on a formula that was not disclosed to the insured, so there was no way to determine what the coverage would be ahead of time. The record, over several years, has been dismal. Most of the time, the insurance company has refused any reimbursement at all, citing some technical issue that is rarely made clear on the laughably named "explanation of benefits" form, laughable because it explains very little and there are so few benefits. When we appealed we sometimes got $55 back, leaving us with a bill of $220. Sometimes we would get a bit more, $80, or $110. And sometimes we would get nothing at all. After the appeals, the reimbursement sometimes changed, and sometimes did not. It was impossible to determine what we should be getting, and whether the insurance company was observing its own policies. Requests for reimbursement were frequently "lost." The company regularly admitted it had made mistakes, but it never seemed to learn from those mistakes.

Occasionally things would run smoothly for a while, and then the company I worked for would decide to change insurers. The new company, which knew nothing of the history of Alex's or Alicia's treatment, would begin, once again, denying all claims. We would begin, once again, to appeal, and to find out how much reimbursement we might expect under the new insurer. This was chaos, and it consumed huge amounts of time. Corporations that think they are saving money when they choose managed care plans might do well to try to determine how much of the company's time

employees are wasting on the phone to insurance companies, trying to get proper reimbursement.

These problems are well known to anyone who deals
with insurance companies, but they are far worse for families
dealing with mental illness. From 1988 to 1998, managed
care plans cut the amount of money they were spending on
psychiatric care by 55 percent, while the reduction in spending on all other medical conditions was 12 percent, according
to Dr. Paul S. Appelbaum of the University of Massachusetts
Medical School. The insurance industry has done this by
establishing separate plans for mental health care, so-called
carveouts that manage only psychiatric care. In 1993, carveouts covered 70.4 million Americans. By 2000, 170 million
Americans were covered by mental health carveouts, which
meant that insurance companies had readily available means
to provide lower reimbursement for mental health care than
for other medical care.

The industry argues that mental health care costs would
skyrocket if psychiatric ailments were covered at the same
rate as other diseases. In a time of rising health care costs,
we, as a nation, cannot afford to boost mental health care
coverage. Fair enough; health care costs are rising, and that
issue must be addressed. But how about some alternative
proposals? If we need to single out one class of illnesses to
save money, why not single out something else? Lower the
reimbursement for heart attacks in people who are over-
weight or who smoke. Let's cut insurance reimbursements
for anyone over sixty-five, because they are not likely to live
long in any case. Let's eliminate coverage for lung cancer,
which is almost always fatal in any case; why throw money
down that hole? Not one of these proposals makes any sense.
Nor does it make any sense to single out psychiatric illnesses
for second-class treatment. Children with cancer receive far

more generous hospital coverage than children with depression and bipolar disorder. Is that fair? Roland Sturm, a senior economist at the RAND Corporation, the southern California think tank, has calculated that providing equal coverage for mental health care, under a managed care system, would add at most 1 percent to employers' health care costs.

No discussion of insurance problems would be complete without noting one more fact. As of 2003, some 43 million Americans had no health insurance at all. That figure includes many children with mental illness, most of whom get no care—none.

Alicia began her classes at Ridgewood High School with wonderful enthusiasm. She sought permission to attend advanced English and arts classes, for which she clearly had the aptitude. I was delighted to see her excited about school, and I was optimistic that she would do well there. I hoped her success would, in turn, improve her self-image, and lead her far from the emotional state she had been in when she'd been cutting herself and attempting suicide. She joined the track team, something she'd talked about for a long time. It was an auspicious beginning.

But within a few weeks, she started falling behind. She skipped class frequently. She wasn't doing homework. She was often out of the house, unsupervised, on school nights. I didn't know whether she was using drugs or drinking, but she was clearly failing in school. She stuck with track for a while, but she had resumed smoking as soon as she returned from Devereux, and she wasn't able to keep up with the other runners. She eventually quit. By spring, it was clear that she would not survive at Ridgewood High School.

In May, at the suggestion of her counselor, she transferred out of the high school and began attending a therapeutic school nearby. Alicia was opposed to the move, but there wasn't much she could say. It was clear, even to her, that something had to change. The school, like Devereux, was entirely inadequate for her academically, but she received far more supervision there, and she regularly attended group therapy. But she missed a lot of classes at this school, too. She refused to get out of bed in the morning. And now her school nights were entirely free, because she rarely had homework. When she did, she could easily get it done on the bus going to or from school. I called her often in the evenings, and she was rarely home. She didn't answer her cell phone. I left messages, and she didn't return them. We saw each other once or twice a week, but I have no idea how she spent her time when we were not together.

During the summer, Alicia made another appeal to return to Ridgewood High School for her sophomore year. I continued to be torn about what was best for her. The therapeutic schools were doing nothing for her academically. She had essentially missed her entire freshman year, and she probably should have repeated it, but what was the point, if she was going to schools that posed little or no academic challenge? Whether she was a freshman again at a therapeutic school, or a sophomore, she wasn't going to learn much. I told her that I would support her return to Ridgewood High School if she would sign a contract with a dozen or so provisions. They included requiring her to go directly home after school, to stay home on school nights, and to do her homework. She would have to attend class regularly. She would have to participate in extracurricular activities, something I thought would keep her busy at critical otherwise unsupervised times and would also give her the opportunity to find new interests. Alicia agreed to sign the contract. I faxed a copy of it to the woman who ran the special education department at the Ridgewood schools. She agreed to meet with Alicia during the summer to make a decision.

The woman was impressed with Alicia's intelligence, warmth, and sophistication. And she was impressed by the contract. On the basis of a single interview, she decided that Alicia could return to Ridgewood High School in September. The news came as a surprise to Alicia's counselor there, who was off for the summer and found out when she returned in September. It came as a surprise to the therapeutic school Alicia had been attending, too, where a place was being held for her in September.

But in September, Alicia refused to sign the contract we'd discussed, or to abide by its provisions. She would handle school the way she wanted to, she said. It wasn't really up to me to tell her what to do on school nights. I felt I'd been duped. She had used the contract to win readmission to the high school, and now she was discarding it. It was then too late to put her back in the therapeutic school, but I would have done that if I could.

Alicia began the year as a sophomore, although she had had none of the preparation her peers had had the previous year. She was intelligent enough to jump into sophomore English and math, and capable of doing well. But she fell back into the habits she'd developed during her first few months there. She skipped classes frequently, at least several times a week, and regularly missed entire days. She did little homework. She didn't run track or participate in any other school activities. She didn't see her psychiatrist regularly, and she wasn't getting therapy or taking any medication.

She was adrift again, as far as I could tell. I worried that in weeks, or months, she would drift into the dark well of depression again. What was to prevent it? There was no way to know whether she was drinking or using drugs, but plenty of reason to suspect she was. I didn't know how she was spending her time, who she was spending time with, or whether she was in any kind of precarious circumstances.

Just before school started, Alicia gave me yet another reason to be concerned. To cap off her defiance, she decided it was time to stop taking her antidepressants. She felt fine and didn't need them, she said. And she didn't need a doctor to tell her so.

Alicia was not seeing a therapist at the time, so she was doubly at risk for a recurrence of her illness. The best treatment for mental illness is a combination of drugs, to ease symptoms, and psychotherapy, to get at the underlying social and psychological causes of the disorders.

Drugs have provided a vast amount of relief for children with psychiatric ailments. Yet the causes of depression, bipolar disorder, schizophrenia, and other psychiatric diseases are unknown. And so very little is known about how psychiatric medications work—even newer, widely used drugs such as Paxil and Ritalin, which are being given to millions of American children and adults. No one knows, either, exactly what these drugs' long-term side effects might be. Nor can psychiatrists say with any confidence who will benefit from them. There is no question that they are helping some of the millions of people taking them, but all of these drugs are used on a trial-and-error basis. It's never clear whether a drug will help, so doctors give one, wait a while, and then try another. And so it goes, as psychiatrists mix various drugs into a cocktail, adding and subtracting until they find a blend that works. The results can be dramatic, as when Alex was switched to a cocktail that included Depakote. But, sadly, this haphazard, scattershot approach to treatment is likely to be successful only in the hands of the most talented and best informed psychiatrists. And success often comes only after years of misdiagnosis and inappropriate or harmful treatments.

Because Alicia was living with Liz, I had no say in whether she should be supervised after school, whether she should be required to do her homework before going out, or whether she should be encouraged to participate in after-school activities. During the marriage, I had often *felt* powerless when it came to the children, because of the explosive disagreements between Liz and me over how to raise them. Now I *was* powerless. I could only watch Alicia fail, watch her waste her time in school; I couldn't do anything about it. If she was bound for another episode of depression, I would have to watch it happen.

Alex and Alicia got along well, and occasionally the two of them would have a long talk, late at night, about what they had gone through. "Alex is so wise," Alicia told me once, after he had counseled her on how to deal with her illness and her friends. Mostly, however, they kept some distance from each other. Their illnesses were different, and their experiences were different. They both had been hospitalized at Four Winds, but they didn't like to talk about that, with each other or with me. It was something they wanted to put as far behind them as they could.

During Alicia's worst years, Alex was reasonably healthy. The miraculous improvement in his condition that had occurred after the treatment by Psychiatrist No. 7 had continued. The worst of his mood swings were kept in check by the medication. But he had missed so much school, as a result of the illness and hospitalizations, that he was far behind many of his classmates, and he struggled.

As I look back at those months, when Alicia was sick, it's difficult to fill in the details about Alex. When one child is in crisis, that child draws all of the family's resources and attention. We had been fighting to save Alicia, who had tried to kill herself more than once. Alex seemed okay, so we focused on her. The reverse had happened when Alex was sick: he got all the attention, and we hoped the others would be all right while we tried to help him. I don't know how we could possibly have coped if Alex and Alicia had both slipped into a crisis at the same time; it was not something I ever had time to think about. The idle thoughts, the concerns about what might happen in the future, came later, when each crisis was past. Struggling with a child in a crisis is a wonderful way to stay in the moment, "in the here and the now," as the Buddhist monk Thich Nhat Hanh puts it. With each crisis, Alex had his time, and Alicia had hers. Matt, who was not diagnosed with a mental illness, was never hospitalized, and did well in school, and took care of himself, didn't have his time. While he was in high school and college, our attention was often rigidly fixed on either Alex or Alicia. During those years, Matt increasingly kept his private life and thoughts to himself, and he nurtured an explosive, unpredictable anger, much of it directed against Liz and me. He distanced himself from Alex and Alicia, and he distanced himself from us. That distance remains.

As the fall progressed, Alicia missed more and more classes. Ridgewood High School allows students to leave the campus whenever they choose. Alicia and her friends often walked into town for lunch and spent the afternoon there, skipping the rest of the day's classes. Even when they didn't,

Alicia often skipped the last class of the day, sometimes the last two. That not only set her back in school, it left her with even more unsupervised time.

At the same time, Alicia had developed a serious, chronic stomach ailment. She was missing morning classes because she would wake up vomiting. She often missed the entire day. Liz took her to the doctor, who couldn't find anything wrong. The illness would come and go, but it continued to be a problem for months. Alicia said it wasn't her fault that she was missing so many classes; she was sick. The stomach ailment didn't explain skipped afternoons, or the classes skipped late in the day. But it was responsible for some of her absences. Often, she would come to school, get sick, then run to the nurse's office in the middle of the morning, and be sent home. I wondered whether the stomach ailment might be a manifestation of recurrent depression. Alicia had been off her medication since the previous summer. Maybe her mood was starting to slide again. Or maybe it was simpler than that. Maybe she'd found an easy way to avoid school. Maybe she was having trouble dealing with her friends again. Maybe she was afraid she would fail in school, and she was trying to avoid facing that. I didn't know what it was.

Liz took her to see the psychiatrist. He insisted that she resume taking medication. This time he prescribed Lexapro, a newer and more expensive version of Celexa. But Alicia's stomach troubles continued. In the spring, we had another meeting with Alicia's counselor at school. With input from the psychiatrist, we devised a different plan. She would continue to be given added leeway in terms of her absences, but she would be more closely supervised when she claimed to be sick. Every time Alicia got sick in school, she would go to the nurse's office until the nurse determined whether she could go home. If Alicia felt better after fifteen or twenty minutes, she would be sent back to class. If not, she would go home. Liz would take her to the doctor and send Alicia back to school the next day with a note. If she did not return with a note, the classes would be considered cuts, not absences due to illness. The idea was to try to sort out whether Alicia was trying to manipulate the system, or whether she was suffering from some yet-to-be-diagnosed physical ailment. We agreed to meet again in a month to see whether things had improved.

At our next meeting, nothing had changed. Alicia was still missing classes, and she wasn't going to the nurse. And Liz hadn't taken her to the doctor, so there were no doctor's notes. The counselor had had enough. There will be no more excuses for getting sick, she said. When you miss a class, it will be counted against you, whether it was because you skipped it or because you were sick. No exceptions.

Within a week or two, Alicia's illness disappeared. It was never a problem again. We never found out what it was, whether it had been stress-related or whether Alicia was somehow making it happen, perhaps not entirely con- sciously. Because of the way it disappeared when Alicia's counselor decided to handle it differently, it seems that it must have been a physical expression of some emotional dif- ficulty related to school. I've asked Alicia about it, and she can't explain it either.

By the time Alicia's stomach ailment disappeared, she'd missed so many classes she was in danger of losing the year. She did lose credit for some half-year classes, and she was in danger of the same happening with science, English, and math. Her accumulated absences added up to the equivalent of six or seven weeks of school. Even so, Alicia was getting Bs and Cs and the occasional A. But because of the absences, she would probably have to repeat her sophomore year.

We discussed a special school once again. One problem was that there was no guarantee Alicia's attendance would be any better. She could skip the bus to a special school as easily as she could skip classes at Ridgewood High School. Another problem, as had been the case with Alex, was that there was no school appropriate for her. We could find no school aimed at kids who are bright but have emotional and behavioral problems, a category that probably includes hundreds of kids in Ridgewood alone.

Liz, Alicia's counselor, and I met with Alicia to tell her the only thing we could think of. We were putting the responsibility on her. She would stay in the high school. If she attended all the rest of her classes, she might, just might, be able to move on to her junior year. Skip any more classes, we told her, and you're a sophomore again. She looked down at her lap. "Okay," she whispered. She didn't argue. She just stood up, grabbed her backpack, and went back to class.

lex's breakthrough with the psychiatrist at Columbia came in the fall of 1999, when he was a freshman at Ridgewood High School. After missing most of the last couple of months of eighth grade, he had started the year with high hopes. He wanted to bury his checkered school record and begin again. I thought he could do it. He was a year older, a little more mature, and he had the new environment to inspire him. Alex began the year in regular classes—history, math, biology, health, and English. But by the end of the first quarter, he was failing most of them. We all knew he was capable of doing the work, but the high school teachers were accustomed to pushing students pretty hard, and the added pressure was too much. As his academic performance suffered, so did his moods.

During the second semester, a few months after he had started treatment with Depakote, Alex was placed in a special education program, in which classes advanced at a slower pace and he received extra help from his teachers. His grades improved to Bs and Cs, but he continued to struggle. He was working hard on his recovery, and that took most of the energy he would otherwise have devoted to school. "Alex's mood plays a major role in how he produces work," his counselor wrote. "He is often very hard on himself, and can get very negative about his future." Alex was the brightest student in the special education classes, his teachers wrote, and he made valuable contributions to class discussions. But none of us—teachers, counselors, parents, or doctors—knew how to help him cope with both his illness and the challenges at school.

The only regular extracurricular activity that Alex showed interest in at the high school was football, and that had ended quickly and painfully, with the coach's bizarre inability to get Alex a helmet that fit. Alex did occasionally go to the school in the evening to help with the music-review show Matt produced and hosted for the high school television station. The one activity that really interested him outside of school was playing the drums. Matt had pulled together a couple of friends to form a group that had the makings of a decent rock band. Matt sang and played guitar. One friend played guitar and another played bass. But they needed a drummer, and Alex had started playing the drums several years earlier, after briefly taking piano lessons. Matt asked Alex to join the band. Alex quickly fell in with the older kids in the band and became friends with most of Matt's friends. For the next two years, before Matt left for college, the band rehearsed regularly and played from time to time in a battle of the bands or at the high school. Occasionally Matt and Alex would clash, but mostly they got along well. Matt would often take Alex along when he met his friends for pizza or a movie.

Alex was bored by the special education classes. One day that spring, he walked into his counselor's office and demanded to be put back into regular classes. She put him into the regular English class. That was all she could schedule in midsemester, but he asked her to put him entirely in regular classes for the following year. The counselor was becoming impatient with Alex's frequent schedule changes; she agreed, but told him he would have to keep that schedule for the year. There would be no more changes. Alex agreed. A month later, just before his freshman year ended, he changed his mind. He talked about dropping out of school altogether. He was fifteen, due to turn sixteen in the fall, when he could be legally entitled to make that decision himself. "He seems to vacillate from day to day . . . in his desire to succeed," the counselor wrote. He was having trouble making decisions in school. One day, he wanted to take a heavier academic load, and the next he wanted to drop out of school. A week later, he would change his mind again.

With the Depakote, Alex's moods improved markedly. He was far more stable, more communicative, happier. But something still wasn't right. It was hard to know whether Alex's difficulties in school were related to his illness, or whether he simply did not want to do the work needed to get decent grades. Mood disorders are so closely intertwined with the identities and personalities of the people they afflict that it's hard to know where the illness stops and the person begins. How much responsibility did Alex bear for his failures in school? The answer mattered, because it governed how he should be treated. If he was having trouble concentrating and reading because of his illness or the medication he was taking, his psychiatrist could help with that. And he deserved special consideration in school. If, on the other hand, he wasn't reading because he'd rather hang out with friends in town, or play video games, he ought to suffer the consequences. It was impossible to know which of these scenarios was right. Maybe both things were happening. Maybe the extra difficulties related to his illness were enough to make him decide that he couldn't do well, so the hell with it.

Alex continued to do well on the medication prescribed by Psychiatrist No. 7. He told me later that he could feel himself becoming agitated from time to time, and he could feel his moods surge upward or downward, but never to the point at which he lost control. Perhaps that was enough, however, to distract him from his schoolwork. He talked about having difficulty concentrating, especially when he was reading. When Psychiatrist No. 7 reviewed Alex's school testing records, he found some evidence of a visual learning disability that might affect Alex's ability to understand material written on the blackboard. The school's testing had revealed this potential problem, but the school psychologist had apparently missed the finding when he reviewed the test results. Alex's counselor arranged for him to be given copies of all notes that teachers wrote on the blackboard. But no system was put into place to make sure that happened. For a week or two, he was given copies of some notes in a couple of his classes, but that effort quickly fell apart.

Alex was skipping classes regularly and making no effort to conceal the fact. He didn't sneak away from campus; he went to the cafeteria, almost always at the center of a group of kids. "When he is out of the classroom," his counselor wrote, "his mood appears to be very good." His illness seemed to be under control, but his life was still unsettled.

I worried that Alex wasn't going to be prepared for college when the time came. Certainly, he was bright and capable enough to do well in college, but he wouldn't have that option if he had any more years like this one. "Don't you understand what you're doing?" I asked him, trying not to let the conversation spin out of control. "Do you want to be pumping gas for the rest of your life, or delivering pizza? If you don't finish high school, you are going to have very few options. And it will be much harder to finish high school later."

I didn't know whether to push harder, or to give him the time and space to work this out for himself. Alex's counselor wasn't much help. She didn't know what to do, either.

Alex began his sophomore year the same way he had begun his freshman year, with ringing enthusiasm and high hopes. He was convinced that he would do better, and he stopped talking about dropping out of high school. He began the year in regular classes. Now, however, he bore the burden of learning, a few weeks before school started, that his parents were going to get divorced. Alex seemed to be suffering from one blow after another. He failed English in the first quarter and received incompletes in all of his other classes. He made up some missed work and turned the incomplete in science into a D, and the incomplete in math, surprisingly, into a B. The talent for math that he'd shown in grade school was still there.

His counselor, who was running out of options for him, decided to put him in a work-study program, in which he would attend classes in the mornings and work in the afternoons. For some students, the motivation and discipline needed to hold a job carried over into schoolwork. At the time, Alex had just started a job he liked at a neighborhood deli. The deli had a policy against facial piercings among employees, and Alex had a ring in his left eyebrow. But the manager let Alex and the other high school kids take their facial jewelry out when they came to work, leave it in the employees' bathroom, and put it back in when they got off work. Alex brought us cold cuts and chicken pot pies and other goodies, which he got at a discount, or sometimes as a gift. For reasons I never entirely understood, the deli job did not qualify for the work-study program, so Alex was forced to quit. The school, which was supposed to arrange for a job, lined up something at a box factory a couple of towns away, but it was too far for Alex to get to by bicycle, and he was still too young to drive. The work-study program was a spectacular failure. He went to school until eleven A.M., and that was it. He had an enormous amount of time on his hands, and his schoolwork did not improve.

Alex asked to be switched back into the regular curriculum for the spring of his sophomore year. His counselor warned him that all these changes would leave him seriously short of credit-hours, and that he might not be able to graduate at the end of four years with the rest of his class. He began having trouble sleeping again. He missed morning classes. And he resumed skipping classes. He had lost many of his friends in the eighth grade because of the rumors about his marijuana use. So he had made friends with older kids whose parents hadn't heard the rumors. Many of those friends were now in the spring of their last high school year and afflicted with "senioritis." Having been accepted to college, they decided that they had given high school about all they were going to give it. Each year in the spring, the high school administration sends a warning letter to seniors, reminding them that college admissions can be rescinded if their grades slip too far. Later, Alex recognized that he had senioritis in his sophomore year. When his older buddies decided to skip school and go to the beach, he went along.

As well as being bored by the special education classes, Alex found them disturbing. Few of the kids, he told me, had any interest in learning. They would run around the classroom, throwing paper airplanes, talking to one another, and, in short, creating an atmosphere in which learning was nearly impossible. "The teachers don't do anything," Alex said. They had long ago given up trying to maintain order, he believed, so very little teaching took place. That was one reason he was skipping classes, and I couldn't blame him. At the same time, however, he was falling further behind with each passing week.

There seemed to be no place for Alex at Ridgewood High School. He needed extra help, but he didn't need to be put in classrooms with kids who had no interest in school. He was bright and curious; with the right instruction, he could easily have done well. But despite the school's sterling reputation, it apparently had no place for bright kids who needed extra help. There were provisions for kids with handicaps and serious learning disorders, but no place for kids who might be in a rocky emotional state, but who were bright and capable of learning.

During the last quarter of his sophomore year, Alex started to feel better about school. He began to focus on his work. His teachers continued to note that he had above-average potential. He made valuable contributions to class discussions, they said, in those classes restrained enough to allow discussion. He worked hard for a time, but he didn't have the endurance to keep at it for more than a few weeks. And he was so far behind, it would have taken a monumental effort to catch up. Alex was in a difficult position. It's not surprising that he felt defeated.

Nevertheless, he continued to make the effort. He began his junior year with a different attitude. He wanted to go to college, and he knew time was running out. He had to get good grades during his junior year. It was time to turn things around, or he would have no choice but the local community college, the last refuge of Ridgewood kids who couldn't get into a four-year college right away. Many of them got jobs so they could buy cars, and both the jobs and the cars distracted them from school. I don't think too many of them made the jump to four-year colleges.

But something had happened to Alex over the summer. He found a new determination. During the fall of his junior year, he gradually, steadily, pulled himself up to the point at which he was earning Bs and Cs in most of his subjects, and sometimes As. He was still easily frustrated, still sometimes lacked the patience to struggle when he needed to. And he often blamed his teachers when he was having trouble. But he kept at it.

I asked him, later, what he thought had happened to help him turn things around. "That's a big question," he said. "I don't know. It just kinda happened. I was hanging out with older kids, and by the time I was halfway through high school, they were getting into colleges. I saw them leaving, and then I started thinking, I want to be with them, I want to be in that same position. I just decided that if I was going to get into college I had to turn everything around." At the same time that some of his friends were leaving for school, others were staying in Ridgewood, in circumstances that Alex didn't find appealing. "I saw a lot of kids sitting around. There are kids I worry about that haven't gone to college. I was like, wow, I can see the paths, I can see what the possibilities are, because my friends are older. So I decided to start working harder. And it was pretty easy. And then it felt good, getting good grades again. I just started working."

This new resolve came at a time when Alex faced many disruptions in his personal life, many of them connected to the escalating arguments between Liz and me over the divorce negotiations.

One such disruption occurred just a few days before he began his junior year. He and Matt were helping me clean out the house I'd rented in Ridgewood. I'd given up trying to encourage the children to spend part of their time at my house. It wasn't going to happen. I was moving into New York, into the apartment of the woman I had now been seeing since the end of the previous year. Matt had been home from college for a couple of weeks—we were now speaking again—and during that time tension had evidently been building between him and Alex.

We were in the basement of my house, packing. The two of them were talking, saying something I couldn't hear. Then I heard one of them say, "I've been waiting for this all week. Come on!" They started hitting each other, hard. They tumbled against the concrete walls, the furnace, and some sharp-edged metal shelves against one wall. Alex had Matt in a head lock, and I had to hit him to break them apart. Though they'd been at it only a few seconds, that had been enough time for both of them to draw blood. Alex turned, screamed something at me, and stalked out, slamming the door behind him so hard that it broke. He walked to his mother's house. When he showed up there, Liz assumed that I had attacked Alex. She put him in the car, drove him back to my house, and ran in the front door, waving her finger at me, saying "What did you do to him? What did you do to him?" She threatened to call the police. "Get the fuck out," I said. Wary of being drawn further into the confrontation, I went down to the basement so I missed seeing what was happening outside: Alex and Matt had encountered each other and started to fight again, on the front lawn. When Matt came down to the basement, blood was trickling from his scalp, dripping down his face, and soaking into his white T-shirt. Alex, I found out later, had taken a blow to the eye hard enough to knock out the silver ring he wore in his eyebrow.

I took Matt upstairs and told him to get in the shower.

Before he did, two police cars pulled up in front of the house. I explained what had happened. They asked me to go inside and get Matt. When he came out, they shifted their focus to him. They didn't seem completely happy with his explanation. They looked at me suspiciously. While we were talking, I heard a radio call in one of the patrol cars. An officer was asking for help regarding an alleged assault by a husband. Then he gave Liz's address.

The police left, apparently not realizing I was the husband in question. I called Liz's house to try to talk to Alex. I got the answering machine. I called a second time. Liz picked up, and said, "Just a minute." A policeman got on the phone and told me not to "keep calling here," or I would face a domestic violence charge.

I hung up. It was deeply unsettling. He was talking to me as if I were a criminal; I could hear it in his voice. I wasn't sure what I could be charged with; I spent the rest of the day worrying that Liz would persuade the police that I had beaten the kids, or that I had threatened her. Later that day, Alex and Matt explained to the police that my only involvement was to break them up, and that I was no threat to their mother. Matt moved in with a friend, and left for college two days later.

The police urged Liz to arrange therapy for Alex, to help him deal with the florid anger he had displayed that day. She set him up with a social worker, who saw Alex two days later. After their appointment, the social worker left an urgent message on my answering machine. I met him the next day. "Alex is in a very, very bad place, and at great risk of hurting himself," the therapist said. A few days later, he called again and asked to meet with Liz and me.

Alex, he told us, was in the grip of "a very serious addiction to marijuana." Marijuana isn't normally thought of as addictive, but the social worker believed that Alex had a serious psychological dependence on it, something that went beyond even heavy recreational use. He employed it as a sort of self-medication. "It doesn't even make him feel good," the therapist said. "It just makes him feel less bad." Alex was still struggling with the divorce, and with a deep concern about Liz's well-being after the divorce. Despite the improvements in his grades and his performance in school, he did not feel he was doing everything he needed to do to get his life together, the therapist said. These were situations "too painful to think about," he said, and "marijuana was indeed very helpful to him in coping with these pains." But the marijuana provided only short-term help, and it was impeding Alex's efforts to get a grip on himself. Weekly visits with me won't break the cycle, the social worker said. And an outpatient drug treatment won't do it, either. After a day or two, Alex was likely to refuse to go. He should be in a full-time substance-abuse program; the social worker had arranged for him to be admitted that night.

This was a lot to absorb in fifteen minutes. I wasn't surprised that Alex had dabbled in drugs, but I had no idea that he was so heavily involved. It was a shock. The social worker suggested we bring Alex in, confront him on the marijuana use, and tell him that he was bound for a drug-abuse treatment program that night.

I agreed. Liz didn't. "He seems so positive lately," she said. The therapist tried to persuade Liz that it was essential that Alex get help. If anything happens to him, the therapist said, you'll have a hole in your life that will never, never go away. He frightened me. Liz shrugged it off. An inpatient program is too harsh, she said. He needs time to adjust to this, to work on it himself. At last the social worker suggested, instead, that we confront Alex anyway, to get the issue on the table for discussion. He called Alex into the room, sat him down, and said, "Alex, how long have you been a heavy pothead?"

Alex was outraged. He had told the social worker about his marijuana use in confidence; he demanded to know why his privacy had been violated. It was a volatile situation, and I wasn't sure where it was heading. Alex's anger was out of control. I was afraid of what he might do. At the same time, I felt some sympathy for him. Discussions with therapists and psychiatrists *are* supposed to be private. Had the therapist been wrong to tell us? But if he hadn't, how would we know Alex needed help? Alex said that his drug use was his business, and it was up to him to decide when he would stop. There was no way he would ever submit to a drug-treatment program. The therapy was over. The social worker wrote, later, that he had several further conversations with Liz and me, but "it was clear that the mutual parental determination to force this issue was not yet in place." That is, Liz still didn't think Alex needed treatment. I did. We were once again at an impasse.

In the days afterward, I had an insistent, recurring daydream, which came to me when I was walking to work, or making dinner, or buying the newspaper. It was a powerful vision and seemed as real as dreams do at night, even though I wasn't sleeping. In this daydream, I was at a funeral. A neighborhood kid had died in a car crash while driving drunk. I didn't know who it was. But in the dream, I could see the church, and the people inside, and a closed coffin. I walked inside. It was time for the eulogy, and suddenly I was the one standing at the podium. I was supposed to speak. Why would I be speaking, unless . . . unless the kid in the casket was my kid? Was it Alex? Had something happened to Alex? I never found out; the reverie ended there. And when it came to me, each time, I was in the church again, and I was at the podium, wondering, with growing terror, who was in the casket.

It was a deeply disturbing thing to experience, more disturbing each time it recurred. I knew it was some distorted manifestation of my worries about Alex. After all we had gone through, when it looked as though he was getting back on track, and doing better in school, we now had another huge problem to address. My subconscious was transforming Alex's drug problem into something far worse, and that was happening, I think, because I felt there was nothing more that I could do for him. Without his mother's agreement, I couldn't get him into a drug-treatment program. We were at the end of some chapter, and I couldn't see beyond that, couldn't see where the story was headed. I was lost.

We didn't discuss Alex's drug use with him again until several months later, in February, when a police car pulled up in front of Liz's house. A lieutenant whom we knew from past incidents in which Alex or Alicia had needed emergency care told Alex that he'd heard that Alex was dealing drugs. Alex denied it. He accused Liz of calling the police on him. The police officer asked Alex to give him anything he had in the house. Alex went up to his room and came down with several empty baggies and a pipe. That's all, Alex told him. I don't have any drugs here. This is a warning, the lieutenant said. If you're dealing, we're going to pick you up. If you're not dealing, it's time you stopped using and got yourself cleaned up.

The sight of a policeman walking away with a pipe finally persuaded Liz that Alex needed drug treatment. She made an appointment for him with a drug rehab counselor, who met with him several times over the course of a month or so. The counselor didn't think Alex was making progress, and she, too, suggested that he be put into a full-time program. But she didn't have any recommendations.

I called her. How was it possible that she treated kids for drug problems, but she didn't know where to send them if the outpatient treatment wasn't working? I would have thought this was a situation that came up all the time. The counselor hesitated, thought for a bit, and finally came up with a couple of possibilities. I called both. One had discontinued its adolescent substance-abuse program years before. The other wasn't right for Alex. I talked to therapists, and to Alex's psychiatrist. None knew what to do. I called the social worker who had confronted Alex about his marijuana use. He had planned to send Alex back to Four Winds, but Four Winds told me that it didn't have a drug-abuse program. There was no resource guide to check, no good source of information on drug-treatment programs that I could find, on the Internet or off.

I was learning something new about bipolar disorder. Many studies have shown a close link between drug and alcohol use and bipolar disorder. The Washington University psychiatrist Barbara Geller tells therapists, "If you see substance abuse, suspect bipolar, and if you see bipolar, suspect substance abuse." When Alex's therapist said that Alex was using drugs not to feel good, but simply to feel less bad, he had identified a central concern in kids with bipolar disorder. They don't use alcohol and drugs for recreation. These kids are often trying to medicate themselves, even if they're being treated with lithium or Depakote. And when they do use illicit drugs, they're risking further damage to a brain and central nervous system already made brittle by the ups and downs of their disorder.

There may be a genetic link between alcoholism and bipolar disorder. That is, some of the same genes that contribute to one might also play a role in the other. But that has not yet been established, Geller says. What is clear is that alcoholism is more common in adults with bipolar disorder than in other adults. But whether the link is genetic or environmental, or both, is not yet clear.

I didn't know about the close association between bipolar disorder and drug and alcohol abuse until after Alex's problems became apparent. I'm not sure I could have done anything to prevent his drug use even if I had known the risk. Alex would have fought any effort to supervise him more closely, and anything I tried to do to establish limits would undoubtedly have been undermined by the conflicts that Liz and I brought to every situation.

From then on, Alex didn't do much to conceal his marijuana use. I don't know whether he smoked at Liz's house, but he left little doubt that he was smoking every day. He has talked about how it calmed and relaxed him.

I didn't think Alex could quit without spending time in an inpatient drug-treatment program. I tried to talk to him, suggesting that he try the treatment, to see whether it would help. The visit from the police had frightened him: "They are watching me, and they won't get off my back." I told him that he needed to be able to show them that he had done something to try to deal with his problem. If they came by again, and he'd made no effort to get help, they might not be so lenient.

But that wasn't Alex's only motivator. Six months earlier, he had received a phone call one day at home. A friend of his had been using drugs the night before, with several other kids Alex knew. After the other kids left, Alex's friend got into his car and drove to Paterson, New Jersey, a tough, crumbling city about five minutes from Ridgewood. Once known as Silk City, for the principal product of its textile mills, Paterson was one of the first industrial cities in America, and it was a thriving community. But in recent decades, Paterson, like so many other cities, had fallen into deep disrepair, physically and socially. And drugs were as easy to buy there as they are in some of New York City's ugliest neighborhoods. Alex's friend, alone in Paterson in the early hours of the morning, found someone selling heroin. The next morning, his parents called up to his room. Time to get up, they said. There was no answer. They went into his room and found him in bed. They shook him, and he didn't move. He had overdosed on the heroin. He was dead.

After several weeks of calling everyone I could think of to find a drug-treatment program for Alex, one of his former therapists recommended a place called Sunrise House, in western New Jersey, that would be covered by my insurance. The coverage was considerably more generous for substance-abuse treatment than it was for mental health, perhaps because the influence of alcoholism on workers' productivity is clearer to management than the influence of mental illness. Under my plan, the lifetime cap for hospital coverage for mental illness was ninety days, most of those being covered at a rate of only 70 percent. But substance-abuse treatment was fully covered for an unlimited number of days.

On March 4, a month after the visit from the police, Alex agreed to drive out to Sunrise House with Liz to take a look at the place. The instructions were simple: He should bring a week's worth of clothes, no aerosol cans, no cologne, no cosmetics that might contain alcohol, no Q-tips, no food, no candy. A portable CD player was okay, but CDs would have to be approved; neither gangsta rap nor anything with violent or drug-related lyrics was allowed. Alex packed a bag according to the instructions, but he refused to agree to enter the program until he got a look at the place. It was located in an old monastery on a hill in a scenic section of western New Jersey, not far from the Appalachian Trail. After brief interviews with the admissions evaluators, Alex agreed to give it a try. A picture taken for his records shows a grim-faced boy, with dark eyes, who looks both angry and frightened. Liz left Alex, and drove home.

At his admission, Alex told the interviewer that he had been smoking marijuana for four years, since he was thirteen. During most of that time, he smoked daily, sometimes two or three times a day. He had occasionally used cocaine, hallucinogens, mushrooms, Percocet, and codeine tablets, all of which were readily available in Ridgewood. And he was smoking a pack of cigarettes a day. He drank only occasionally, and then rarely enough to become intoxicated, he said.

The next evening, Liz attended a patient-family group therapy meeting. After the session, Alex became angry and said he couldn't stand the treatment. He wanted out immediately, and he pleaded with Liz to take him home. Liz was ready to put him in the car. Alex's agitation was understandable. It was the first day in years in which he hadn't smoked marijuana or had a cigarette. Whatever else was happening at Sunrise House, that alone would have left him agitated and anxious.

Liz called me when she got home, to say she was going to go out and bring Alex home the next day. "Under no circumstances should you bring him home," I said. "We've had to work for months to get him into treatment, and if we give up now, we'll never get him back there. He's gone through the worst of it. Each day ought to get easier." I did everything I could to impress on Liz the importance of continuing his treatment, but I was failing. She agreed, finally, not to do anything until we had a chance to talk to his counselor the next day.

The next morning, I spoke to Alex's counselor. Alex was still agitated, still demanding to go home, and had threatened to throw a chair during a group session in the morning. Now the staff psychologist was considering discharging him. The psychologist was concerned that Alex might do something to hurt the staff or the other patients. I pleaded with the counselor not to discharge him. "He says he's suicidal, which he's not," she said. She explained that Alex was in what they call the transition period, which sounded to me like withdrawal. Alex knew that his mother was on the verge of coming to pick him up, she said. "He knows his mother is just waiting for a call." She asked me to talk to Liz, and said that it was important that I persuade her to give Alex what she called a bottom line. That is, a flat refusal to take him out of the program. I called the psychologist and persuaded him to give Alex one more chance. I thought Alex would calm down as soon as he understood that his parents agreed that he could not come home yet. The psychologist was skeptical but agreed to wait until that evening. I doubted that Liz and I could agree on keeping Alex in the program, but I had to try. I called her again and told her that she would be doing Alex grave harm if she took him out of the program. When I hung up, I didn't know what she was going to do.

Alex spoke to both of us, separately, that night. His mother held firm. He hung up on her and called me. "Dad, you have to get me out of here. This is my last chance. I fucked up my phone call with Mom. It's like jail, I can't stand it here." It ripped me apart to hear him ask for help, and to tell him that I couldn't help him the way he wanted me to. "You're there to get better," I said. "You have to give it a week or two before you know whether it's helping." I told him I would talk to him the next day, and we said good-bye. When I put down the phone, I started to cry.

After he'd spoken to both of us, Alex spent some time with his counselor again, under the eye of the psychologist. He slowly calmed down, and went to bed. The next morning, he plunged into the program with enthusiasm. If he was going to be stuck there, he told me later, he thought he might as well see what it was all about. His strategy shifted. The quickest way out, he decided, was to participate as vigorously as possible.

He spent eighteen days at Sunrise House, and his mood lifted dramatically as the days passed. Visits were limited to one hour on Sunday afternoon. Liz and I split the hour and visited separately; we split attendance at the weekly parent-child group therapy sessions, too. The sessions were different from the many I had attended in hospitals and with the kids' therapists. Therapists were listeners; the Sunrise House counselors were taskmasters. They did most of the talking. They educated the patients about drug abuse, and they talked about the kind of support that the kids would need when they got out if they were going to stay clean. They used exercises to encourage communication between parents and their children.

One night, they gave us sentences to complete—for instance, "I feel (blank) when my (son) (daughter) uses drugs." These were gimmicky, and unlike anything I'd seen in therapy, but they often prompted valuable discussions. We talked about Alex's unwillingness to spend an occasional night at my apartment in New York. I had decided that our relationship was so far gone that he just didn't want to spend any time with me. I tried to see him once a week in Ridgewood, but given the complexities of his social calendar, we got together only once or twice a month for dinner. I tried to get him to visit me at the apartment in New York City. I told him to bring a friend or two, to crash on the couch and the floor. He mostly cooked dinner for himself at Liz's house, and he had a couple of recipes he wanted to make for me. But he only managed to get into the city about once every four or five months. The reason, he explained, was that he couldn't go a day without marijuana, and there was no place in New York that he could go to discreetly light a joint. Also, he knew about the tough drug laws in New York State. Whatever other problems his heavy drug use was causing, it had been cutting deeply into the time he and I could spend together. He said he looked forward to spending the week-end with me as soon as he finished the program.

I picked Alex up the day he was discharged. His mood was lighter and his face brighter and happier than at any time since before he got sick. We stopped for McDonald's ham-burgers and fries on the way home, as an antidote to the food at Sunrise House, which he had hated. Alex went back to school with bright prospects. It was a memorable day.

Alex was to attend an intensive outpatient drug program for some weeks after his discharge. He was to go to the pro-gram four days a week after school, and stay for several hours. The idea was to keep him away from friends who were using drugs, and it would give the lessons he'd learned at Sunrise House time to solidify. He began the sessions the Monday after his discharge, but after a couple of days, he decided he didn't need it. Liz acquiesced. It was too hard for her to force Alex to do anything.

A year later, I asked Alex about Sunrise House. His impression was entirely different from mine. "Sunrise told me that I was weak, that I was pathetic, that I couldn't do anything without them," he said. "They told me that weed was stronger than I was, that it had a stronger hold over me than anything, and I just laughed. I'm not doing cocaine, I'm not shooting heroin. Let's keep things in perspective."

While he was at Sunrise House, he had attended meetings of Narcotics Anonymous. For a short time after he dropped out of the outpatient treatment program, he went to NA meetings, sometimes with a friend. He found the program useless. "There are maybe one or two people in those meetings who actually care and want to make their lives better," he said. "The rest of them are there for the free coffee and doughnuts, I'm sure. My friend and I used to go to NA to meet girls." He also went to Alcoholics Anonymous meetings a few times after he left Sunrise House, he said, and he found them equally worthless. "We'd go around the circle and say how long we'd been sober. I'd say how many days I'd been sober, and some guy would say twenty minutes, or forty-five minutes. He drove to the meeting from a bar."

Three months after Alex left Sunrise House, it became clear to me that he was using drugs again. I called his counselor at Sunrise House to ask what I could do. She was disappointed to learn that he hadn't gone to the outpatient program she'd set up for him, and said I should try to get him enrolled there again. She thought it would be difficult for him, and probably not appropriate, to return to Sunrise House. If the outpatient treatment failed, however, he would have no alternative but to reenter it or enter some other inpatient program. But without Liz's cooperation, I couldn't do anything.

During Alex's stay at Sunrise House, Liz had decided she needed a few days away. The stress of the situation was getting to her. She left for a long weekend to visit her parents in Florida. Liz said she had provided for Alicia to stay with friends and their parents while she was away. Liz left on a Friday. That night, Alicia was to be at her friend Jessica's house, with Jessica and her father, and she was supposed to call me when she got there. I didn't hear from her, so I called early in the evening to make sure everything was fine. There was no answer at Jessica's house. I tried again several times, and there was still no answer. My phone rang around nine o'clock. It was Alicia, telling me that she was at Jessica's house. My caller ID showed otherwise. "You're home," I said. "I can see it on my phone. What are you doing there?"

"We're headed to Jessica's right now," she said. "Her father is picking us up." I told her to call me as soon as Jessica's father arrived. I waited a half-hour. There was no answer at Jessica's, or at Liz's. I left a message at Liz's, and Alicia called back a few minutes later. I asked to speak to Jessica's father. A man got on the phone and said, yes, Alicia was with him, and everything was fine. He seemed confused when I told him I thought the girls were supposed to have been with him much earlier. As soon as I hung up, I realized I'd been had. That wasn't Jessica's father; it was one of Alicia's friends. It would take me more than an hour to get the car out of the parking lot in Manhattan and drive to Ridgewood. I called the Ridgewood police and asked whether they would check the house for me.

Two hours later, a policeman called back. Alicia was at the station. She'd been in the house with Jessica and half a dozen friends, most of whom had scattered out the back door when he pulled up in front. He had found empty beer bottles, marijuana, and a pipe.

I drove out to pick up Alicia. We got back to my apartment about three A.M., and she spent the weekend with me. Siblings were not allowed to visit at Sunrise House, so when I went out to see Alex she sat in the car while I went inside. I didn't take my eyes off her until her mother got back from Florida and I took her back to Ridgewood. To my mind, this was cause for severely restricting her social activities for a while, until she could earn back the trust she had so blatantly violated. Liz grounded Alicia for a few days, but quickly tired of the effort. Alicia was once again roaming through town after school, visiting friends that we had never met, and, in all likelihood, drinking again. As my therapist had told me over and over again, there was nothing I could do about it.

Alex got and lost half a dozen jobs during the last couple of years of high school. He'd decide that he couldn't work on weekend nights, because that was when he spent time with his friends. Or he couldn't work for a boss who didn't respect him and treat him the way he thought he should be treated. Or he didn't make enough money; he was going to quit and look for a better job. He wanted a car badly, and he knew that neither Liz nor I had the money to buy him one. But even that wasn't enough to help him keep a job. He wasn't sure whether he wanted an old junker that he could buy for a few hundred bucks, or whether he should save a few thousand dollars for a decent used car. He finally did go for a junker, a Ford Escort he picked up for $800. The shocks were bad, the electrical system was held together with duct tape, and the brakes were nearly gone. It lasted for a few months, and then the electrical system went out. The car was dead, and it would cost more than a thousand dollars to fix. Without a new electrical system, it wasn't worth anything. Alex had the car taken away. He had lost all of his investment, and his bank account was near zero.

During the rest of Alex's senior year, his improvement in school continued. His grades were Bs and Cs. But he never did acknowledge that it was the school's job to set rules, and his job to follow them. From the time he had threatened to drop out, his counselor had decided that it was best to go easy on Alex, to try to keep him in school, and he had been exempted from the school's policies on attendance. During his junior and senior years, he accumulated so many absences that if he had been held to school policies, he wouldn't have been promoted either year. In hindsight, I think it was a mistake to have relaxed the rules for Alex. He had learned to push until adults gave in. His approach in high school was to follow the rules when he chose, and ignore them the rest of the time.

Yet despite his mixed feelings about school, Alex developed warm relationships with several of his teachers. One inspired him to think about a career teaching in high school. Others encouraged him to pursue his interests in history and photography. On the last day of school, his English teacher made no attempt to hold class. She sat quietly at her desk while the students talked and joked among themselves. She was retiring, so this would be her last day in the classroom. Alex spent the entire period sitting with her, talking about what she was going to do when she left school, and wishing her well. He was also extraordinarily well liked by the other students, including those who had graduated a year or two ahead of him. He had more friends than I could keep track of. I came to think of him as the unofficial mayor of Ridgewood; we couldn't go anywhere in town where Alex wasn't stopped on the street, hailed by friends from passing cars, and greeted by people in restaurants and coffee shops. I asked him how he had managed that. "I'm a peacemaker. I'm friends with everybody," he said. "My thing is, I can't rely on myself too much in bad situations." He said he worried that he would be at a party or with a group of kids and would unpredictably "go off," as he put it, becoming angry and unable to control himself. "So I rely on my friends. They will be at my back, and I'll be at their backs."

Alex has never tried to hide his illness from his friends. And he never seems to worry too much about what anyone thinks. But lately he has had some reservations about that. "Bipolar disorder" has become a mock term of derision among kids in Ridgewood, he said. When a kid is a little too rowdy, someone will say, "What are you, bipolar?" Or, "At least you're not bipolar."

"People have said that to me," Alex told me. "They have actually said that to me." And he thinks to himself, "Well, yeah. I am."

"What do you do?" I asked him.

"I just shake my head and walk away."

Like many people who take lithium or Depakote, Alex has a noticeable hand tremor, a side effect of the drugs. "The other day, someone asked me why my hand shakes, and that was the first time I didn't want to say I was bipolar. I just said, I'm on medicine, so leave it at that. More often than not, I like to shock people, and have them say, 'Wait a minute, you seem halfway sane, how are you bipolar? How are you getting along? How are you working if you're bipolar?' That's what people say to me. But this time, I didn't want to let people know. Because people think differently about me."

Not long ago, I asked him whether his emotions were still a problem for him. As far as I could tell, he was doing well on Depakote. But, from his point of view, he wasn't doing well enough. He becomes angry in front of his friends, he said. On a couple of occasions, he found himself at a party where Brian—the young man who had raped Alicia—was also a guest. On those occasions, Alex found it difficult to control himself. He blames that partly on his illness. Maybe it is the illness, in part; I don't know. But who among us wouldn't have trouble remaining in control in the same situation, confronted by someone who had sexually assaulted a sister?

During the fall of his senior year, Alex continued to think about college. He took the SATs, and met some of the college recruiters who came to Ridgewood, but he couldn't decide where he wanted to go. He didn't fill out any applications. After Christmas, he was still thinking about college, but I thought it was too late. Most colleges require that applications be submitted by February 1 or thereabouts, and Alex was not going to make that deadline. But he found a number of colleges that had rolling admissions and accepted students as late as the spring of their senior year. Alex had friends in college in northern Vermont. One weekend, we drove up there to take a look at some of the schools he'd found that interested him. He applied to two of them, and was accepted at both. Without help from anyone, he had pursued a goal I thought had already eluded him, and he had found a college that seemed perfect for him. It was an important step for him, proof that he could take control of his life. He had rescued himself from near disaster in high school, and he had found a college that recognized his achievement and was eager to have him.

When the Ridgewood High School students gathered in June on the football field for their graduation, Alex stood proudly among them. Four years after he had wordlessly watched Matt graduate on that field, he did what his brother had done. He was one of the most popular and best-liked students in his class.

Alex had turned his illness into an asset. He knew what was important to him, and he was learning how to get it. All of this had seemed so improbable only two years before, when he had talked of dropping out of high school. It was a wonderful moment. I was fiercely proud of what he had accomplished.

In the final weeks of that school year, just before Alex's graduation, Alicia was facing the ultimatum that we had given her in her counselor's office. She would no longer be penalized for cutting classes; we could think of no way to encourage or force her to attend. But if she continued to miss classes, we had told her, she would repeat her sophomore year. If she stopped missing classes, she would be a junior the following year.

Skipping classes was not Alicia's only problem. In the spring of her sophomore year, just before we gave her the ultimatum in school, she was picked up by a Ridgewood policeman who saw her walking down the street with a twenty-one-year-old man, carrying two six-packs of beer, which they hadn't bothered to hide inside a paper bag. The man had taken her to a liquor store and bought the beer for Alicia and her friends. It was a simple matter for the police officer to conclude that something was amiss. To complicate matters further, Alicia made a few flip remarks to the policeman, putting herself at risk of further trouble in addition to a charge of possessing alcohol.

The police officer filed a complaint. Alicia's case was referred to a probation officer in the county courthouse in Hackensack, a few miles from Ridgewood. I didn't learn of any of this until I received a notice to attend a meeting with the probation officer. A few weeks later, Liz, Alicia, and I sat down together with the probation officer, a tough, smart young woman who immediately assumed control of the situation.

"What do you expect will happen to you here?" she asked Alicia.

"I don't know, I thought maybe I'd get a period of adjustment," Alicia said. I looked at her. What on earth was a "period of adjustment"? And how did Alicia know about it? The probation officer wondered the same thing, and she asked Alicia about it. "I don't know, a lot of my friends have had periods of adjustment," Alicia said. Some had been on probation, too. Who exactly had she been spending time with? Some of her friends, she said, had been picked up for possession of alcohol or drugs. She knew some who had been sent away to rehab programs. The probation officer explained that a "period of adjustment" was a lighter form of probation, in which kids who are arrested need to perform certain tasks before their cases are closed. That was not what the probation officer had in mind for Alicia, however. What she ordered was something less: Alicia's case was held open for 180 days, during which time she had to write a letter of apology to the policeman who had stopped her, observe six hours of municipal court proceedings in Ridgewood and write a report on her visits, and write a three- or four-page essay discussing her arrest and what she thought it meant.

As it happened, the arrest more or less coincided with an improvement in Alicia's behavior. She did what the probation officer had ordered. Six months later I received a notification from a New Jersey judge that her case had been dismissed. From the day that we gave her an ultimatum in school, she stopped cutting classes. She got credit for all of her courses, without any relaxation of the attendance requirements. It was a dramatic change; until that day, she had not made it through a week without missing a class since the previous November. It seemed that Alicia, like Alex, had found a way to turn things around. She got good grades, despite missing so many classes earlier in the year, and earned warm praise from her teachers. It was a triumph. For the first time, we started to talk about college.

Alicia began her junior year in September 2003, much the same way. She attended classes regularly, and she was getting As and Bs. She wasn't terribly excited about the work, though, and she said some of her classes were a waste of time. She had started seeing a therapist weekly during the summer, but she stopped in October. "I just didn't want to deal with it," she said. But she continued to go to class, to do her homework, and to keep her grades up. Once again, I encouraged her to take advantage of some of the extracurricular activities at the school, but she showed little interest. I was confident, however, in a way I had not been only a few months earlier, that she would finish high school and go on to college, where she would have every opportunity to do well.

Alex started college that same September, with great excitement. He was happy to be out of the house, the scene of so much conflict between his mother and me, and, more recently, between him and Matt, who had just graduated from college and was living at home while he looked for a job. Alex and I sat down together during the summer to talk about what classes he might want to take. He made his decisions and sent in his registration materials.

The semester began auspiciously. For his first writing assignment, he wrote about an experience he'd had with a few friends one night when he was in high school. They were driving in a friend's Camaro, a "muscle car," when they happened upon a pack of illegal street racers in a parking lot. It was two A.M. The lot was near a lonely stretch of highway in southern New Jersey. Alex and his friends signaled to the others that they wanted to race. Several cars followed them, and the race was on. Alex and his friends reached a speed of 175 miles an hour and won the race easily. For his writing assignment, he wrote about the experience of traveling at that speed, the fear, the exhilaration, and the happy sense of relief when the race was over. His writing teacher asked him to read the piece to the class; his fellow students gave him a round of applause when he finished. I cringed when I read the essay: this was the first I'd heard of the race. But it was well written. I applauded him, too.

For another class, he wrote a paper that was, in part, about having bipolar disorder. It was entitled, "Who Am I?"

"Although this disorder does not define me as a person, it affects every aspect of my life, almost all of the time," he wrote. But "there is much more to me than this illness. I love writing and the outdoors. I personally feel that the greatest high you can get is when someone tells you that you have helped them. Seeing a person go from a depressing state of mind at the beginning of a conversation to a great big, comforting smile at the end makes you feel something so amazing. It is indescribable."

Alex displayed remarkable maturity during those first weeks in college. I was astonished at how much older he looked. He had trouble with a friendly but unruly roommate, so he talked his way into a single room. He quickly found a job. He got himself a late-night talk-and-music show on the college radio station. When I went to visit him in late September, people called out to him everywhere we went. It hadn't taken Alex long to establish himself.

At the same time, however, he was struggling in some of his classes. Ridgewood High School, which had lifted so many requirements for Alex and made so many exceptions for him, had left him unprepared for the demands of college. Reading had always been difficult for him; he had trouble concentrating, he said. He was not adept at taking notes in class, or at organizing and reviewing material before a test.

One night, standing at a counter at one of Alex's favorite hot dog spots in New York, I told him about the first exam I'd taken during my freshman year in college. It was in physics, which was my major. There were six problems on the test; I couldn't answer any one of them. I remembered walking back to the fraternity house where I lived, alone, crying. "But you kept going," he said, before I could supply the punch line. I nodded. He got the point.

That's where the situation stands. Alex has made enormous strides since the worst days of his illness. But, like others his age, he is still searching for his path. I'm optimistic. He is a seeker; I don't think he will settle for less than what he wants. I watch, and wait, and I help when he asks. And I listen to his dreams, and, quietly, I dream my own dreams for him.

Alicia's sudden improvement in school occurred during the end of her sophomore year and the beginning of her junior year. That was just about when Alex began to do well in school, too. Was that an accident, or did it mean something? Their experiences of illness had been quite different. Yet both seemed to improve markedly around the age of sixteen, around the time they were emerging from the worst of the turmoil and confusion of adolescence. Could that have had something to do with their recoveries? I decided to look into it.

Researchers once believed that most of the brain's growth and adaptation after birth occurred during the first few years of life. Newer studies have provided convincing evidence, however, that the brain continues to grow and to change throughout adolescence. The frontal lobes, which play a role in making wise judgments and resisting impulses, do not reach their adult form until about age twenty. The cerebellum, which is involved in social interactions, does not mature until late adolescence. Various other connections are made during adolescence, and levels of the brain chemicals called neurotransmitters, which are involved in signaling between brain cells, also change.

Is it possible that some of the troubles Alicia and Alex experienced were related to these changes in the adolescent brain? And does that explain why, as they got older, they seemed to be doing better? Researchers cannot yet answer those questions, but there is reason to think that psychiatric ailments in children are indeed connected to the neurological changes that occur during adolescence. If that's true, then further study of the developing brain might point the way toward better treatments for Alex, Alicia, and the tens of millions of children who will suffer the same debilitating emotional upsets. The idea that their illnesses are related in part to adolescence was one reason to hope that Alex and Alicia will continue to get better.

I think about that when friends and colleagues ask me, as they often do, how the children are. "Fine," I tell them. "Much better." But I don't say what else I'm thinking. Alex and Alicia *are* fine now, but how long will that last? There have been so many times during the past few years when one of them seemed to be improving, and when I thought things were fine—until suddenly they weren't. If what research suggests about the adolescent brain is correct, it's likely that they will do better from now on. But the knot in the stomach, the tightness in the chest, the fear that their illnesses might suddenly come back, will never go away. There are times when I can take a breath, times when I can relax a little bit. But I can never forget what they have been through. I cannot make the past go away.

CHAPTER NINE

Where are we now? What have we learned from these difficult years?

When I was nearly finished with this book, I sat down with Alex first, then with Matt and Alicia, to conduct something like formal interviews. I needed their help to fill in some of the holes in this story, but more than that, I wanted to know how they felt about all the things we had been through. I wanted to know what Alex and Alicia thought about their illnesses. And I wanted to ask Matt what it was like to grow up with a brother and sister with mental illness. It was an unusual exercise. When I sat them down and turned on the tape recorder, our roles shifted. I became the reporter, and they were the people with a story to tell. They said things to me, as an author and interviewer, that I don't believe they would have told me as their father.

Alex put off the interview for months. He was willing to talk, he said, but he worried that it would upset him. He wasn't sure he wanted to think about all that had happened. I knew what he meant. I had felt that way often while working on this book.

When we finally made time to sit down in my apartment, he spoke with great emotion. He was participating in the book, he said, because he wanted his story told. "I've said to people, 'If you want to understand what I've been through, and why I feel so proud of the way I handle myself now, read my dad's book.' "

Alex remembered having trouble in school as early as the fourth grade. "I just thought I had ADD," he said, "that I was one of those kids with just another learning disorder." (It wasn't a bad guess; Psychiatrist No. 2 had thought the same thing.) But he didn't remember having trouble with his schoolwork. What he remembered was that he behaved strangely and didn't know why. "It was just bad times, doing things I wish I hadn't done. Like having the police come to pick me up, and then running away. I remember treating it like it was a game. I was having so much fun when I was running. I remember running into the woods another time when they came, and I lost my shoes in the mud and just kept running. I didn't understand it. I didn't get it."

When the police took him to the hospital, he remembered kicking the back window of the patrol car, and the metal gate between the front and backseats. Laughing, he said, "I remember I was full-force kicking those windows, and kicking that gate, and I laughed to myself. I thought, Wow, these things can take a lot, they're not breaking. And I thought, All right, I guess I can't cause any havoc in here. Then they took me out, with all the guys holding me down. And when you have people holding you down, that doesn't make you comply." He fought harder.

At school, the principal had given him his own room, an

office next door, where he could go when he was upset, to calm down. He was the only one in the school who had that privilege. "All right," he remembered thinking, "I know I'm screwed up." What made it worse was that his teachers didn't seem to know any more than he did about why he was behaving strangely. "Everything freaked them out. They didn't understand it. They thought I was so much crazier than I am. Everybody thinks I'm crazier than I am. They don't understand that medication can actually tame these things, and that you can live with it." In middle school, there was one teacher who had shown particular empathy for him. She told him he could come and talk to her any time. Later, she told her own son, who was Alex's age, that she didn't want him to play with Alex. "It was just such a two-faced thing," Alex recalled. "To say, 'Oh yeah, I'll help you with your problems,' and then, 'As soon as he starts hanging out with my son, I don't want to have to deal with him anymore.'"

He remembered excelling in math when he was younger, but with the advent of his illness, he began to lose interest in schoolwork. "As soon as I started having emotional problems, people were doubting me, and then I doubted everything. I decided not to care about my work. I thought all the cool kids failed. I honestly thought that. The nerds do well, and the cool kids and football players get Cs and Ds. I ended up not doing anything." Did that have anything to do with his illness? "No, it was just trying to fit in. I had to fit in, because I was so screwed up, I didn't know where I fit."

Alex didn't think his hospital stays had done anything for him. I thought the hospitals had helped at least by providing some structure and setting clear limits, but that wasn't it, he told me. He hated them and wanted to get out as quickly as possible, and he knew that following the rules was the way to do that. The first time he was hospitalized, he was told that his roommate had shot someone. "Why am I in here," he told me he wondered, "when I ran away from school, and this kid shot someone? The first thought that went through my head was, I shouldn't be here. I'm not like this."

The next time he was admitted, "I remember waking up next to a kid, and he introduced himself. I said, 'Why are you in here?' And he said, 'I shot myself in the head.' That was that. I didn't feel there was anybody like me there. The only reason I stopped lashing out was because I was afraid to go to those hospitals. I remember, as soon as I started becoming chill with the kids, they all seemed to open up, and they were telling me where hidden razor blades were, where there were chemicals, and aerosol cans to sniff, whatever you needed. People wouldn't take their medicine, they would put it on the back of their tongues, and then they'd keep it and sell it for food. It was like prison. That's what scared me. I didn't deserve to be in prison. I don't want to live with the fact that I've been to a place that has white padded walls. I saw things that nobody should see. I saw a kid, a karate expert, taking on twenty guards. There was blood, broken bones. It was horrible. And I remember him getting strapped down in the same thing I saw on Hannibal Lecter [the serial killer in the movie *The Silence of the Lambs*]. He had a cage over his face. They put him in the back of a white, unmarked van, and drove away. If that's not scary, I don't know what is."

Alex has thought a lot about what it means to have bipolar disorder, and about how it affects him. "I don't know what bipolar is or what it does, but when I don't take my medicine, I do more crazy things than when I do take my medicine. And when I take my medicine, I can live my life. And I know

I'm going to have to take it for the rest of my life. That's all I know. I've never had a therapist who's helped me work through my problems. The only thing I have is the psychiatrist who gives me pills to solve my problems. Believe me, I'm not against taking medication. But when I go away, I sometimes forget my medication. And by the fourth day, I can feel it starting to come on. I feel myself getting angrier, very stressed and anxious and nervous, and all these crazy emotions. I can feel it seep in."

When Alex feels bad, he likes to get away, to be alone with nature somewhere. "I'll sit in a field, and watch the trees blow in the wind, and that is all I need to get me by. You can find the beauty in everything. Even the simplest things. Watch the dew run down a leaf. This world really is amazing. I can always go for a walk, just by myself, just to listen to the wind. I can sit on the beach. There's nothing like sitting on the beach. There's a vast expanse of water, and I'm sitting at the edge. It's thousands of miles before there's another piece of land. And it's all being controlled by the pull of the moon. You think about stuff like that, and you say, 'Wow, I'm a part of this.' It's just nice."

It seemed easy for Alex to talk about his experiences with bipolar disorder, because it is something he thinks about every day. Alicia, who was sixteen when we talked, spoke about her experiences with depression in a very different way, as if that chapter in her life had been closed. She had a hard time remembering what had happened, what she had felt, how she had coped.

When I asked Alicia where the story began, she started with Alex, and the troubles he was having in school. "He would be taken out in handcuffs, and I was nine years old and everybody was asking why my brother was being taken out in handcuffs. And I had no idea." When Alex was taken to the emergency room on what the kids knew to be National Pot Smokers' Day, she took some heat about her brother being a drug dealer. "Some kid wouldn't stop talking about why he got arrested. So I flipped out and punched him in the stomach. He never said anything to me again."

Alicia remembered the story of her own illness beginning in sixth grade, when she kissed the boyfriend of a "popular" girl and the kids started baiting her about being a "slut."

The "popular" girl "had a lot of power socially, and she could easily sway people's opinions. So if she said Alicia was a slut, I was a slut. That kind of ruined my entire sixth-grade year." During the summer after sixth grade, Alicia became friends with the girl, for a time. "I had actually become the popular girl, and then I had the social power. And she ended up becoming nobody. That's when that was resolved."

What did she do to cope? She looked for help, and she didn't find any. Not even from Liz and me, who were too busy helping Alex. "He was having more, I don't know what the word is . . . more 'loud' problems. I felt like I had no one to talk to, and no one cared. I didn't really have any friends." She didn't discuss her troubles with her counselor or any other adult. "I was quite a passive person at the time. I didn't want to say anything and call attention to myself. Looking back on it, I was depressed. I don't know if I recognized that at the time." Her first suicide attempt was related to the upheaval at school, she said. "That was my way of saying, 'Fuck you, I don't care what you think about me.' " It was at the beginning of the next year, in the seventh grade, that Alicia started cutting herself.

Liz's first boyfriend was also the father of Sarah, one of

Alicia's closest friends. It wasn't an easy friendship, however. "Sarah is a possessive, controlling friend. I was forced to be with her all the time, with our parents' dating. It was constant. One time, I got into a fight with her, and she ended up cutting herself. And her father called me up and started yelling at me and saying it was my fault. And I said, 'Look, it's not my fault your daughter has emotional problems. I've been in that situation, and it's nobody else's fault. I don't care what you say, you can't blame me for this.' And then he ended up breaking up with Mom because of it. Then I got a guilt trip from her, about something that was totally, completely, not my fault."

Alicia was coping with all of this while also trying to sort out her complicated relationship with David, her discovery of sex, the unpredictable, unstable social situation at school, the rape, and her parents' divorce. It's hard to imagine how anyone could have gone through all that without suffering from depression and making bad choices.

Because so much had been forced upon her, she began reflexively to fight back whenever she was told what to do. "I tend to rebel against authority," she said. She doesn't like to be told what to do by her parents, by teachers at school, or, when she's had part-time jobs, by her supervisors and employers. She said she'd been talking to her therapist about this. "I have two extremes. I have a passive extreme, where I'm not going to say anything, and I'm going to smile and be polite and nice. Eventually the passive thing leads to rebellion, and that's when I freak out and lose my job or get kicked out of school. I need to find an in-between place where I can be assertive without being rude, polite but saying what I need to say."

Alicia's view of hospitalization was different from Alex's.

She didn't see the hospitals as prisons. She just thought they were a waste of time. "I went repeatedly, and it didn't help me, because the short time period does nothing. It's like, 'Hey, I think I might be starting to get better,' and then you go back home, and you see a therapist once a week, and you have no one to talk to again, and it's like, 'What am I going to do?' It might help some people, but it didn't help me."

Now, she said, she feels depressed sometimes, but not to the degree that she did before. "I'm much more in control. I have a lot more knowledge and a lot more help than I did then. I never, ever think about hurting myself. I never think there's no way out, there's nothing I can do. There's never despair that complete and total."

Matt was, by far, the most guarded of the three children. Our relationship had been distant for a long time, and it had grown even more distant since the separation and divorce. He and I shared a taste for odd movies, and when he was in high school we regularly drove into New York to catch something at one of the art houses. Matt never talked much about his classes and rarely shared his feelings. It was difficult to know what he was thinking, about the family, about his future, about Alex and Alicia's illnesses, or about anything. We talked about the news, about politics, about movies and music, but not much about ourselves. When he left for college, he had even less to say about what was going on. I took him to school at the beginning of each year and picked him up at the end, and visited from time to time during the school year, when I could stop over on a business trip. Despite all of those visits, I never met his friends, except for a perfunctory handshake now and then, when we passed somebody he knew on the way into or out of his fraternity house. Matt kept his personal life private.

When we sat down for our interview, I asked Matt what he remembered about the beginnings of Alex's illness. He remembered Alex's first hospitalization and that it had forced cancellation of a car trip to Michigan to visit my parents. Matt was then in the ninth grade. He found Alex's "freak-outs" mysterious. He didn't know what to think about them. "I wasn't sure what was going on," he said. "It was surpris-ing, and disconcerting." But he didn't think of Alex's illness as catastrophic. "I thought these were isolated incidents," he said. "Until I got out of the house and into college, I don't think I realized how abnormal they were." He was never frightened by Alex, he said, "because I thought he would be able to recover from it. And he did recover from it."

Matt remembered a lot of conflict between him and Alex when they were growing up. "When we were really young, I know that our relationship was adversarial. We had to share a room, so we had to deal with it, one way or another. And we didn't deal with all of it. A lot of it was buried underneath the surface. And it would come out, there would be a boiling point from time to time. That would fade away when we both realized we were going to have to deal with each other." Their relationship improved when Alex played drums in the band, Matt thought. "I was the leader of the band, and he knew that I was in charge, so there wasn't much of a conflict. I think it worked out well."

I asked Matt whether Alex's and Alicia's illnesses, and the uncertain outlook for their futures when they were younger, made him feel compelled to succeed, to be the one who did well. "No. Actually, I felt like it was easier to bury myself in my schoolwork than to deal with what was going on. I didn't want to spend a lot of time at home." But he also said that, because he was the healthy one, he'd been burdened with the idea that he should do something to help. "I kind of wondered why this thing that was happening to both of them had skipped me. I felt a little lucky, I guess. . . . I felt like I was an island of stability in what appeared to me to be a very chaotic environment. I did feel like there was more I should have done. It wasn't until later I realized that there wasn't anything I could have done."

It was clear, however, that Matt was conflicted about trying to help. When I asked him about Alex's and Alicia's problems with drugs and alcohol, he did feel there was something he could do. "I've never used a single illegal drug in my life. I don't know what it's like to use something like that; to self-medicate. If I had to deal with the kind of things they've had to deal with, I don't know how I'd respond. I can't blame them, but I can try to lead by example, by not using drugs. I'm not their parent. I can't send them to their rooms if they don't behave. The best I can do is be a role model, and have faith in them that they're going to be able to solve their own problems."

Throughout the interview, Matt made it clear that he was talking to me only to provide some balance in the book, to provide a point of view different from mine. He was not happy that I was writing this book. He wanted to be sure that Alicia and Alex were protected, and that their views were fairly represented. He seemed to be straddling two places. On one hand, he was telling me that he didn't think there was much he could do to help Alex or Alicia. At the same time, though, he was taking a very protective, parental role in trying to protect them from whatever I might say in this book. "As long as it portrays Alex and Alicia in a fair light, and as long as they're comfortable with it, I'm comfortable with it. As far as my own role, I'm much happier to be in the background."

In the course of talking about this book, we did not reach a reconciliation. When we last spoke, he was angry about the book, and still angry about the way the divorce had unfolded. The gulf between us was wider than I had suspected. I don't know whether he and I will be able to bridge that distance. I hope we will one day recover something of the relationship we had when he was younger. But we have a long way to go. "I feel like I really don't have a father figure anymore," Matt said near the end of our interview. It pained me to hear that. And I think it pained him to say it. But I don't know what I can do about it.

As I began the research for this book, I became increasingly aware of the scandalous disregard with which we treat our mentally ill children. Children and adolescents with psychiatric disorders are among the most neglected and mistreated members of our society. Of the millions of American children with emotional problems, only one in five receives any medical care. Some of this is a consequence of poverty; poor children are less likely to receive medical care of any kind. But the problems with mental health care cut across the economic spectrum. Most children with mental health problems are from the middle class, according to a report by the office of the U.S. Surgeon General. The one in five children who does receive treatment might be considered to be one of the lucky few, but the record suggests otherwise. Treatment of children's psychiatric disorders is often abysmal. The diagnosis is missed. The children are given the wrong drugs, or the right drugs in the wrong doses. They are offered little or nothing in the way of counseling and psychotherapy. They are admitted to psychiatric hospitals repeatedly, and discharged under the orders of insurance companies after only a few days or a week, long before a diagnosis can be made or an effective treatment established. Many of the few children receiving care lose it abruptly when their insurance runs out, which happens much sooner for mental illness than it does for diabetes, heart disease, or any other ailment. Some parents are forced to give up their jobs to become full-time care managers for their children. Some lose their jobs, because they can't get their work done while they are being called away to emergency rooms, school classrooms, police stations, hospitals, and juvenile detention centers to attend to their children.

In 1999, the National Alliance for the Mentally Ill conducted a nationwide survey of parents of mentally ill children. Only about half of the children were receiving drugs or medication, and these were families in which the children were known to have a psychiatric ailment. Two thirds of the parents said their pediatricians and primary care doctors did not ask about mental health issues during routine visits. About half said that their children had been denied access to care, or received only limited care, as a result of decisions by their managed care plans. When asked whether school officials had the training to respond appropriately to mental illness in children, only 7 percent said yes. Nearly all of the parents felt shunned by neighbors and friends because of their children's illnesses, and half said they had been blamed for those illnesses.

There are millions of families like these, families convulsed by the torment of their children's mental illness. And few of them have the resources I have. As a reporter, I knew where to find answers when I had questions. I had access to leaders in the fields of psychiatry and psychology. And I had enough money to pay for medical care myself when the insurance company didn't cover it. Few families have the connections I have, and few can afford to pay for psychiatric care that isn't covered by insurance. Their struggles and their suffering, I realized, must be far worse than mine.

They need help, and they don't get it. I've talked to many parents who, frantically in search of care for their children, find they have nowhere to go. Some, unable to pay the high costs of care, are tragically forced to relinquish custody of their children to state welfare agencies, who can then place the children in hospitals or special schools. Often, parents take this desperate step only to find that the state does not provide the care it promised. Even if parents can afford to pay for care, there are too few child psychiatrists and far too few children's psychiatric hospitals. Schools, which are often the first to see the symptoms of mental illness—or should be the first—fail children by turning their backs on the problem, deferring to the health care system or, worse, the juvenile justice system. And few politicians in either the state or the federal government are willing to do anything to improve the situation.

The emotional and financial strains on the family can become unbearable. The children quickly fall behind in school, and their social and emotional growth is crippled by their ailments. As their ability to cope with friends and school fails, some commit suicide. Others are arrested and confined in juvenile detention centers, where "treatment" may consist of little more than handcuffs, rough discipline, and exposure to criminals. The guards are not trained to distinguish healthy juvenile offenders from those whose unlawful behavior might be a symptom of an untreated psychiatric illness, or a bad reaction to medication.

We are failing these parents, and we are failing their children. We need to recognize that this is a public health crisis, and we need to do something about it.

For decades, reports by government agencies, health advocates, and psychiatrists' organizations have pointed to the serious problems in the way America deals with mental illness in children. One of the most recent such reports was issued in the summer of 2003 by a presidential panel called the New Freedom Commission on Mental Health. There is something "terribly wrong, terribly amiss" with the nation's mental health care system, the commission concluded. And the consequences are overwhelming: "When the system fails to deliver the right types and combination of care, the results can be disastrous for our entire nation: school failure, substance abuse, homelessness, minor crime, and incarceration. . . . There are hundreds of thousands of people with serious mental illness in other settings not tailored to meet their needs—in nursing homes, jails and homeless shelters."

None of this is likely to change until parents become as angry and fearless as breast cancer patients or AIDS activists. We must stand up and talk about our children and how they have suffered. There are costs to coming forward. We must acknowledge that something in our own genes might have been partly responsible for our children's illnesses. We must admit that our parenting might have contributed to the illnesses' severity.

We live in a society that still stigmatizes people with mental illnesses. Those of us who come forward and publicly acknowledge that our children have psychiatric ailments walk right into the teeth of that stigma. I've seen it on the faces of people I've spoken to: *If your children are suffering from depression and bipolar disorder, then what is wrong with you? What have you done to them?* Until we are willing to talk about our children and our families publicly, America's tragic failure to care for its mentally ill children will continue. It is up to us; no one else can fight for them as fiercely as we can.

have struggled to find a way to end this story. Books have endings, but life goes on. As long as I am alive, this story will continue for me. As I was completing these last few pages, I awoke one morning at the conclusion of a dream. I was in a house I did not recognize, waiting for Alex to arrive. He was driving a highly unconventional vehicle, a kind of boat, about the size of a pickup truck, that had been modified to travel on land. The weather was bad; it was starting to snow. I wasn't worried about his driving or his judgment, but I was worried that his "boat" might not get good traction on the slippery highway. I stood in front of the house, in the falling snow, looking toward the highway and waiting. A police car pulled up. Frantic, I ran toward the car. The police officer opened the back door and helped Alex out. Alex's vehicle had crashed, but he was fine. I ran to him and hugged him. The strange vehicle, I suspect, represented the unconventional path that Alex has been following. And despite the crash, he arrived safely. Although Alicia was not part of that dream, the same has been true for her. She, too, has followed her own path, and she, too, has arrived safely.

Alex and Alicia have overcome obstacles that most of us will never have to face. During the darkest days of their illness, I kept hoping that their efforts to overcome those obstacles would leave them with something of value, something that would make them wiser, more sensitive, and more aware than they would have been if they'd chanced upon an easier path. There had to be some payback for all the suffering they endured. And there has been. Alex and Alicia are far more understanding and more sensitive to their own feelings and to the feelings of others than they would have been if they had not experienced, and survived, their illnesses. As teenagers, they have learned things about themselves that I did not learn about myself until these past few years, as I traveled beside them.

At the end of *An Unquiet Mind,* Kay Redfield Jamison considers what she would do if she could choose whether or not to have bipolar disorder. If lithium didn't control her illness, she says, she would not choose to have it. "Depression," she writes, "is awful beyond words or sounds or images; I would not go through an extended one again." But lithium does work for her. So: What would she choose? "Strangely enough, I think I would choose to have it. . . . I honestly believe that, as a result of it, I have felt more things, more deeply; had more experiences, more intensely; loved more, and been more loved; laughed more often for having cried more often; appreciated more the springs, for all the winters. . . . I have seen the breadth and depth and width of my mind and heart and seen how frail they both are, and how ultimately unknowable they both are."

I asked Alex and Alicia the same question: If you could have chosen not to have bipolar disorder or depression, what would you have done?

"I feel exactly the way she [Jamison] does," Alex said. "Nobody will ever feel the things I've experienced. There's something amazing about insanity, a lure about it. It's not right, it shouldn't be happening, yet it does. You see things, you hear things, you feel things that aren't right. But after the bad things are over, you realize how amazing it was, what you just went through. When I'm happy . . . nobody can be that happy. Nothing can bring me down. And when I'm depressed, I know it's going to end. I'm manic-depressive. There are two sides of the spectrum, so you can't be at one side forever."

Alicia said she, too, would leave her past unchanged. "It's part of who I am, I think. It's made me, I don't know, unique. I'm not like most of the kids I know. I like that." There is a downside, too, she acknowledged. "I think it's something I'll have to deal with for the rest of my life." I reminded her that her depression had brought her a lot of pain. "And a lot of insight," she said. "I understand people better now. I understand myself better."

When I interviewed Alex and Alicia, four years had passed from the time Kay Jamison signed a copy of her book for Alex, and wrote the inscription "Things will get better." I didn't believe it then. But she was right. Things did get better. I can hope that the worst days are behind us.

If it were my choice to make, I would have chosen easier lives for Alex and Alicia. I'm glad that they have come to terms with their illnesses. And I wouldn't change who they are. My love for them is mixed with enormous admiration for the struggles they've been through, and how they've survived. But they suffered for years. I watched them suffer, and it hurt, and I wish it hadn't happened.

I have little doubt that my failings as a parent, and especially my excessive, misdirected anger, contributed to the severity of Alicia's and Alex's illnesses, and to my troubled relationship with Matt. I failed them. If I'd behaved differently, things might have turned out differently. There is nothing I can do about that now, except to learn from what we have been through, and to treat them differently in the future.

Alex, Alicia, and Matt are not the people they once were. I look forward to watching them become the people they are going to be.

n January 2005, a television critic in the *New York Times* began with this observation: "Mental illness is the new sex." The article went on as if it were dissecting a fashion trend. "Psychological disorders are the next big thing," it said. "Therapy is in the air, in the culture and in everyone's medicine cabinet." On prime-time television, the *Times* said, mental illness "is still just novel enough to incite laughter."

Note the use of the words "psychological disorders." The implication is that mental illnesses are not *real* illnesses; just something in the mind.

As far as I can tell, the article produced no outcry, no angry letters, no criticism in the media. Now, try a thought experiment. Suppose the words "psychological disorders" were replaced with autism or Alzheimer's disease. *Autism is the next big thing. Alzheimer's disease is just funny enough to incite laughter.* Imagine the outcry those statements would produce.

Many people still do not recognize mental illnesses as real illnesses in this country, even though nearly all of us have someone in the family who's been afflicted with a psychiatric disease.

Sadly, the failure to understand psychiatric illnesses extends to the medical profession. For two years, the Food and

Drug Administration, doctors, and the drug industry have struggled to respond to reports that antidepressants might increase the risks of suicide. As the father of two children who have been on and off several different antidepressants during the past decade, I followed the debate closely.

The main thing we've learned is that the research needed to determine conclusively whether antidepressants are help-ful or harmful has not been done. Why? The drug industry is not foolish enough to look for problems with drugs that earn billions of dollars. And the government hasn't done the studies either, because, presumably, it's the drug industry's problem. Nobody has made the study of mental illness in children a national priority. And so we may never know for sure whether antidepressants increase the risk of suicide.

It soon became clear to me, however, that nearly all the risk could be eliminated if doctors used the drugs properly. It's clear that many children and adolescents are helped by antidepressants, and it would be wrong to restrict their use. But most doctors, including many psychiatrists, are using the drugs recklessly—because they offer their patients no follow-up.

That was certainly the case with my children, who were given the drugs and sent home. I was never told to watch for a change in mood, an obvious precaution that all parents should take. No doctor or psychiatrist ever offered to call reg-ularly during the first few weeks my children were on anti-depressants. I was never told to check in. And yet a simple program of regular calls and visits during those first few weeks could probably eliminate almost all of the suicides that occur following the use of antidepressants.

The problem is that pediatricians and family doctors, who spend only a few minutes on each patient visit, don't have the time to do it. Psychiatrists, who charge by the hour, don't get paid for follow-up phone calls. And if a suicide does occur, the medicine and the drug will get the blame, not the doctor who wrote the prescription.

In other words, follow-up would be nice—but there's no money in it.

What's the solution? I'm convinced that only a national healthcare system, responsive to Congress and the voters, would give the public the power to change the way doctors are reimbursed. Under the current system, reimbursement decisions are made by the insurance industry, drug companies, and the American Medical Association. These are not people who have your children's welfare in mind.

It's been one year since the publication of *Acquainted with the Night,* and I'm heartened to report that the book has made some contribution toward calling attention to the problem of mental illness in children.

The response to the book has been overwhelming. I was particularly gratified to hear from fathers. Remember fathers? They are so often left out of discussions about children with mental illness. It always seems to be the mothers who rush home from work, shuttle the children to their therapists and psychiatrists, and are home when the worst and most frightening symptoms of their children's illness appear—the threats, the wild, erratic behavior, the ambulance trips to the emergency room. "My wife was always the one to read, to try to understand and deal with my daughter's illness," one father wrote me. Then he spotted *Acquainted with the Night* in a bookstore. "Something about the title and jacket notes of your book hooked me. I have never read anything before that seemed like it was written about our lives as well. Father to father, I just wanted to tell you that I understand what you went through."

"Your book is my life," one reader wrote. Another said, "As I read your book, I cried. I know there is at least one other person who shares my journey. You have given me some hope." This woman wrote the letter while awaiting a court appearance. She had been held in contempt of court for missing her child's IEP meeting at school.

"The most arduous pages were those in which Raeburn blames his wife and himself for their children's disorders," said a review by Brooke Schewe, Director of Outreach and Development for Families Together in New York State. "He shares his emotions with the reader, emotions I and most families of children with mental health disorders can relate to—guilt, confusion, despair, fear, anxiety, sadness, shame, hopelessness, anger, frustration, and bewilderment, to name a few." Schewe said she'd heard countless such stories from families she's worked with, but that "neither desensitized nor prepared me for such a vivid narrative of everything that can possibly go wrong for a child in need of mental health treatment."

Not all of the responses were so complimentary. "I believe Mr. Raeburn needs classes on parenting," one parent wrote. "His children do not have mental illness—they have a father who is looking for anyone, except himself, to blame for his children's behavior." Such are the perils of writing about one's mistakes, bad judgment, and anger. As I tried to explain in these pages, parents can no more "give" a child a mental illness than they can give a child a brain tumor. Mental illnesses are *real* illnesses. But, as I also acknowledged repeatedly in the book, my years-long struggle to cope with my children's illnesses, and my explosive anger at critical points, increased their suffering. Some readers responded mostly to what I wrote about my dissolving marriage. "As someone participating in a difficult marriage," one wrote, "I am in near total isolation. I can't talk to anyone about it."

In a review in the *Washington Post,* Daphne Uviller wrote that the book was "a searing and eloquent indictment of America's insurance industry that ought to land CEOs in jail. Barring that, *Acquainted with the Night* should reignite the revolution needed to overhaul this nation's approach to health care."

I haven't put any CEOs in jail. And the book hasn't yet ignited that revolution. But I am using every forum I can to call for radical change in our healthcare system. My efforts did receive a response from Senator Susan Collins of Maine and from Representative Henry Waxman of California, who wrote in the January/February 2005 issue of *Health Affairs,* "In documenting his struggles to obtain basic mental health services for his children, Paul Raeburn is ringing an alarm bell for action. Congress and the administration should answer his call."

I hope *Acquainted with the Night* will persuade more parents to stand up, tell their stories, and use their real names. Our children have no advocate but us. Until we stand up for them, and demand better care, they won't get it.

The question I'm asked most often is, "How are your children doing now?" I'm happy to report that the hope with which I ended the book has been fulfilled. Both of them are healthy, their prospects are bright, and I have no doubt that their lives have been deepened and enriched by their struggles to overcome their illnesses. I offer other parents the same profound hope.

Paul Raeburn
New York City
February 2005

ACKNOWLEDGMENTS

When I first thought about writing this book, I wasn't sure how to begin. I needed help, and I found that help at the Carter Center in Atlanta. The center awarded me a mental health journalism fellowship, which gave me the financial support to begin work and the opportunity to discuss it, during an early, tentative stage, with a warm, receptive, and intelligent group of fellows and advisers at the Carter Center, including Mrs. Rosalynn Carter.

In the years since, I have talked to countless parents, children, psychiatrists, researchers, and therapists. They helped give me the confidence I needed to tell my own story, and strengthened my conviction that the stories of mental illness in children need to be told.

I could not have had a better agent for this book than Beth Vesel. Beth helped me to clarify my thoughts about the story I was trying to tell. We worked together for several years. I'm not sure many other agents would have had the patience to stay with me for so long, helping me to get it right. My editor, Gerry Howard, had a profound influence on the shape of this book. Without his contributions, it would have been a very different and much less interesting book. I would also like to thank the staff at the Writers' Room, the wonderful Greenwich Village refuge where I did much of my writing, editing, and rewriting.

Alex and Alicia allowed me to examine thousands of pages of their medical records, school records, and their writing. More important, they allowed me to reveal deeply personal details of our lives together. They have been an inspiration to me, and I hope they will provide the same inspiration to other children, teenagers, and parents who read this book.

Reliving the scenes I've described here was a harrowing experience. There were many, many nights when I felt that I couldn't go on, that I would have to abandon the project. On those nights, my wife, Elizabeth DeVita-Raeburn, would listen, help me understand why I felt the way I did, and guide me to a deeper understanding of the story I was struggling to tell. She read every word of the manuscript—some parts, she read many times—and helped me to sharpen and focus the story. I don't think I could have finished this book without her help, her wisdom, and her love.

BIPOLAR DISORDER AND DEPRESSION

Child & Adolescent Bipolar Foundation
1187 Wilmette Ave., P.M.B. #331,
Wilmette, IL 60091
www.bpkids.org

Juvenile Bipolar Research Foundation
788 Morris-Essex Tpke.
Short Hills, NJ 07078
www.bpchildresearch.org

The Bipolar Child
www.bipolarchild.com

Depression and Bipolar Support Alliance
730 N. Franklin St., Suite 501
Chicago, IL 60610-7224
http://www.dbsalliance.org

The National Alliance for the Mentally Ill (NAMI)
Colonial Place Three
2107 Wilson Blvd., Suite 300
Arlington, VA 22201-3042
www.nami.org

The National Mental Health Association
2001 N. Beauregard St., 12th Floor
Alexandria, VA 22311
http://www.nmha.org

Center for the Advancement of Children's
   Mental Health at Columbia University
1051 Riverside Drive
Columbia/NYSPI Unit 78
New York, NY 10032
www.kidsmentalhealth.org

SUBSTANCE ABUSE

Substance Abuse and Mental Health Services Administration
Room 12-105 Parklawn Building
5600 Fishers Lane
Rockville, MD 20857
www.samhsa.gov

RESEARCH

National Institute of Mental Health (NIMH)
Office of Communications
6001 Executive Blvd., Room 8184, MSC 9663
Bethesda, MD 20892-9663
http://www.nimh.nih.gov

American Psychiatric Association. *Diagnostic and Statistical Manual of Mental Disorders,* 4th ed. Washington, D.C.: American Psychiatric Association, 1994.

Blum, Deborah. *Love at Goon Park: Harry Harlow and the Science of Affection.* New York: Perseus, 2002.

Carter, Rosalynn, with Susan K. Golant. *Helping Someone with Mental Illness: A Compassionate Guide for Family, Friends and Caregivers.* New York: Times Books, 1998.

Dudman, Martha Tod. *Augusta, Gone.* New York: Simon & Schuster, 2001.

Garbarino, James. *Lost Boys: Why Our Sons Turn Violent and How We Can Save Them.* New York: Free Press, 1999.

Gilmore, Mikal. *Shot in the Heart.* New York: Doubleday, 1994.

Hobson, J. Allan, and Leonard, Jonathan A. *Out of Its Mind: Psychiatry in Crisis, a Call for Reform.* Cambridge, Mass.: Perseus, 2001.

Jamison, Kay Redfield. *An Unquiet Mind.* New York: Knopf, 1995.

———. *Night Falls Fast: Understanding Suicide.* New York: Knopf, 1999.

Karr, Mary. *Cherry.* New York: Viking, 2000.

Levenkron, Steven. *Cutting: Understanding and Overcoming Self-Mutilation.* New York: Norton, 1998.

Mondimore, Francis Mark. *Bipolar Disorder: A Guide for Patients and Family.* Baltimore: Johns Hopkins University Press, 1999.

Neugeboren, Jay. *Imagining Robert: My Brother, Madness and Survival, a Memoir.* New York: William Morrow, 1997.

Papolos, Demitri F., and Papolos, Janice. *The Bipolar Child.* New York: Broadway Books, 2002.

Pruitt, David B. *Your Adolescent: Emotional, Behavioral, and Cognitive Development from Early Adolescence Through the Teen Years.* New York: HarperCollins, 1999.

Sheehan, Susan. *Is There No Place on Earth for Me?* New York: Random House, 1982.

Solomon, Andrew. *The Noonday Demon: An Atlas of Depression.* New York: Scribners, 2001.

Steinberg, Marlene, and Schnall, Maxine. *The Stranger in the Mirror: Dissociation, the Hidden Epidemic.* New York: HarperCollins, 2000.

Strauch, Barbara. *The Primal Teen: What the New Discoveries About the Teenage Brain Tell Us About Our Kids.* New York: Doubleday, 2003.

Wolpert, Lewis. *Malignant Sadness: The Anatomy of Depression.* New York: Free Press, 1999.

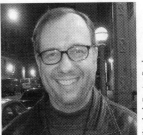
Elizabeth Devita-Raeburn

ABOUT THE AUTHOR

Paul Raeburn was formerly a senior writer and editor at *BusinessWeek,* where he covered science and medicine for seven years. He is the recipient of many distinguished writing awards and is also the author of *Mars: Uncovering the Secrets of the Red Planet* and *The Last Harvest: The Genetic Gamble That Threatens to Destroy American Agriculture.* A native of Detroit, Raeburn lives in New York City with his wife, the writer Elizabeth DeVita-Raeburn.

Printed in the United States
by Baker & Taylor Publisher Services